WATCH YOUR BACK!

A VOLUME IN THE SERIES

The Culture and Politics
of Health Care Work

edited by
Suzanne Gordon and Sioban Nelson

*A list of titles in this series is available at
www.cornellpress.cornell.edu*

WATCH YOUR BACK!

How the Back Pain Industry Is Costing Us More and Giving Us Less—and What You Can Do to Inform and Empower Yourself in Seeking Treatment

RICHARD A. DEYO, MD

ILR Press
an imprint of
Cornell University Press
Ithaca and London

The views expressed by the author of this book are not intended as a substitute for medical advice, diagnosis, or treatment provided by the reader's personal physician.

Copyright © 2014 by Cornell University

First published 2014 by Cornell University Press
Printed in the United States of America

Library of Congress Cataloging-in-Publication Data

Deyo, Richard A., author.
    Watch your back! : how the back pain industry is costing us more and giving us less—and what you can do to inform and empower yourself in seeking treatment / Richard A. Deyo MD.
        pages cm — (Culture and politics of health care work)
    Includes bibliographical references and index.
    ISBN 978-0-8014-5324-3 (cloth : alk. paper)
    1. Backache—Treatment. 2. Back—Diseases—Treatment. I. Title.
II. Series: Culture and politics of health care work.
    RD768.D44   2014
    617.5'6406—dc23   2014006972

Cornell University Press strives to use environmentally responsible suppliers and materials to the fullest extent possible in the publishing of its books. Such materials include vegetable-based, low-VOC inks and acid-free papers that are recycled, totally chlorine-free, or partly composed of nonwood fibers. For further information, visit our website at www.cornellpress.cornell.edu.

Cloth printing   10 9 8 7 6 5 4 3 2 1

To Lynda, Mom, Andy, and Liz:
the lights of my life

CONTENTS

CONTENTS

PREFACE

Back pain is among the most frustrating medical complaints for patients and doctors alike. Both expect the usual medical paradigm of diagnosis and treatment to work as it usually does. That is, we doctors take a medical history, examine the patient, order tests, and figure out exactly what's wrong with the patient: exactly what anatomical structure or physiological disruption is causing the pain. Then we provide the best treatment designed specifically for that problem, and voilà! The patient gets better.

Sadly, this paradigm routinely fails us when it comes to back pain. The pain sometimes goes on well beyond the time it takes tissues to heal from injuries. Patients often don't improve when the doctor thinks they should. Doctors often don't prescribe tests or treatments that patients think they should.

We have MRI scans of the spine that show all manner of abnormal things, but it turns out that pain-free people often show the same things. We have wonderful medications that minimize pain for people with short-term problems but regularly create mischief if they're used for too long. We have a steady stream of new strategies and devices for surgery but little scientific evidence of how effective or safe they may be.

We also have media and marketing that tell people they should always be pain free and that doctors can always cure pain if they just try hard enough. Sometimes the media imply that doctors are holding back on treatments we know to work. If only it were so.

The reality is that no one is pain free all the time. I have a variety of discomforts on a daily basis: shoulder pain, plantar fasciitis, tennis elbow, and yes, often back pain. Headaches when I'm under stress. And doctors have no incentive to hold back on treatments that work. Indeed, they have real incentives to provide treatments whether or not they work. The more we do, the more we're paid.

When I attend professional meetings of doctors interested in back pain, there's always interesting hallway discussion and lively dinner conversation. These discussions are less guarded and more candid than what you read in medical journals and newspapers. Rather than hear only about the best results from the latest treatments, I also hear about the disappointments and disasters. I've often found myself wishing that patients could hear the things I hear when people discuss new gadgets, techniques, or drugs for managing back pain.

There are so many competing approaches to treating back pain that you're very likely to get multiple, sometimes conflicting, recommendations. Back pain is so common that almost anyone can hang out a shingle, claim to have a cure, and make a living. One of the things we'll explore is why so many treatments of dubious value can survive.

But things aren't all as bleak as this may sound. The reality is that there are effective treatments. They don't promise a permanent cure of all back pain, but they offer big improvements and a better quality of life. And they are generally treatments that the patient has within his or her control. The key to improvement is often taking a more active role in decision making and self-care. We'll look at the scientific evidence to support this claim.

Throughout this book, I'm going to use "doctor" as shorthand to refer to health care providers. This term applies to naturopathic physicians and chiropractors as easily as it does to medical doctors. It's more familiar than "provider" to most people outside the health care industry. I mean no slight to the many nurse practitioners, physician assistants, acupuncturists, physical therapists and others who care for patients with back pain on a daily basis. Indeed, many patients consider those providers to be their "doctors." I'll sometimes refer to people with back pain as patients, but of course, they're only patients if they seek health care. Many people with back pain never seek health care and choose not to become patients. But terms such as "consumer," or "customer," or "client" seem to turn patients into purely financial entities: people who simply buy services rather than people who are struggling with illness.

People with persistent pain may not be as objective in their thinking as those without. They're thrust into a labyrinth of unfamiliar medical terms and clinical services. They need compassion as well as pills or procedures, and they're ultimately quite different from people who are shopping for a car or for home insurance.

Ultimately, this book isn't about miracle cures. It's about having people with back pain take more control of clinical decisions and more control over their own well-being. I hope to empower you and reassure you about a common, but maddening, part of life.

ACKNOWLEDGMENTS

I've had a lot of help over many years in shaping the ideas presented here. They are a result of experience with patients but also of research work, discussions, and debates with too many people to credit individually. But I thank my many colleagues at Oregon Health and Science University, the University of Washington, the University of Texas Health Science Center at San Antonio, Dartmouth Medical School, Keele University in England, the Vrije University in Amsterdam, the Group Health Cooperative in Seattle, the Kaiser Northwest Center for Health Research, and elsewhere for their knowledge, wisdom, and inspiration.

Special thanks are due to General David Fridovich and Dr. Jerome Groopman, who graciously agreed to interviews for this book and who have been courageous and candid in describing their experiences with back pain. Special thanks also to colleagues who read and offered critical feedback on parts of the book. They improved both the thinking and the writing. These include Beverly Hallberg, Floyd Skloot, Mark Schoene, Judy Turner, Jerry Jarvik, Linda Pinsky, Jim Rainville, John Saultz, and Dan Cherkin.

Some other Seattle and Portland colleagues have for years stretched my thinking. Two surgeons, John Loeser and Stan Bigos, are among them, as is Janna Friedly. So are Michael Von Korff and Karen Sherman, both at Group Health Cooperative, and Roger Chou at Oregon Health and Science University.

Two former University of Washington colleagues, Sohail Mirza and Brook Martin, are now at Dartmouth, along with longtime colleague Jim Weinstein. They've been among my most energetic, thoughtful, and helpful colleagues. Dartmouth's Jack Wennberg introduced me to geographic variations in care and the notion of shared decision-making. Other New Englanders who shaped my thinking are Bob Keller, Steve Atlas, Al Mulley, and Jon Lurie. Gary Schwitzer has sensitized me to the importance of the media and to its common shortcomings. The ongoing collaboration of all these individuals is something I prize.

Among the early influences in my career were two European orthopedic surgeons: Gordon Waddell and the late Alf Nachemson. Several other international colleagues also exerted a major impact on my ideas. Rachelle Buchbinder and Mary Wyatt from Down Under have demonstrated the value of population interventions and challenged conventional wisdom. Peter Croft, Martin Roland, Nadine Foster, Kate Dunn, Martin Underwood, and their UK colleagues have taught me how to measure treatment effects, to estimate prognosis, and much more. Bart Koes, Raymond Ostelo, Lex Bouter, and Maurits Van Tulder have sent scientific rigor and clear thinking from the Netherlands. Canadians Michele Battié and Claire Bombardier have championed influential genetic studies and growth of the Cochrane Collaboration, respectively. Among others, Aage Indahl of Norway demonstrated to me the benefits of exercise and restraint in other interventions.

The contributions of these interviewees and colleagues shouldn't be read as endorsements, but they deserve credit for much of what's good in this book. The points of view and opinions presented here are mine, and I'm responsible for anything that isn't so good.

I'm extremely grateful for the opportunity to work on a project that I find so interesting and important, one that is also a bit of a departure from the usual scientific research and publication process. Thanks for the opportunity are due to the Department of Family Medicine at

Oregon Health and Science University and my department chair, Dr. John Saultz.

Suzanne Gordon, the series editor at Cornell University Press, offered valuable suggestions, persistent support, and important enthusiasm. Thanks to her for seeing something promising in the original proposal.

Finally, it seems pro forma to thank one's spouse or partner in an acknowledgment. But this thank you is way more than pro forma. My wife, Lynda, read and offered insightful edits to every chapter. She often forced me to say things more clearly and to expunge silly academic or medical jargon. She helped keep me honest. Perhaps most important, she provided support and encouragement when I had doubts about the feasibility or wisdom of the project. She is my most precious partner in every way.

WATCH YOUR BACK!

Chapter 1

BACK PAIN NATION

Since nearly all of us get back pain, you may be one of the sufferers. If you're not, you probably will be. Two-thirds of adults report back pain at some time in their lives. Think of it as a frustrating part of a normal, healthy life.

Yet back pain is distracting, debilitating, or disabling for some people. It's among the leading causes of work disability, and it restricts many people's activities. Compared with cancer, diabetes, or heart disease, back pain may seem trivial to some, but it's costing our society nearly as much as these life-threatening conditions.

If you have back pain, you're confronted with a growing menu of treatments that are rapidly increasing in use. When our research team at the University of Washington scrutinized the growth in treatments for back pain, the numbers were startling. Over roughly a decade, from 1994 to 2005, there was a 300 percent increase in MRI scans of the low back for Medicare patients. There was over a 100 percent increase in the use of narcotic painkillers for back pain and over a 200 percent increase in spinal fusion surgery. Expenditures for epidural steroid injections in the Medicare population—thanks to increasing use and rising prices—increased over 600 percent. We'll explain and examine these treatments later.

These numbers mean that someone was making plenty of money from back pain. But as we'll see, there's no sign that, on average, patients were getting better results over this time. These changes reflected a booming back business.

How much do we spend on back pain? Coming up with realistic cost estimates is a challenge. One approach is to ask how much more people who have back pain spend for medical care than similar people who don't. Our research group's best estimate, based on national surveys: $86 billion in 2005. That was 9 percent of *all* health care costs, comparable to the costs of cancer or diabetes. And that figure didn't even consider the costs of work loss or disability compensation.

Our team also found that costs for back pain were increasing faster than costs for medical care overall. And, of course, overall medical costs have increased faster than general inflation for many years.

Market watchers estimate that spinal implants alone—the plates, screws, and gadgets often used in spinal fusion surgery—cost $3.8 billion in 2009. That's not counting the hospital charges or doctors' bills. The national hospital bill for those operations—which includes the gadgets— was around $38 billion, although hospitals collect less. Drug market analysts estimated the market for narcotic painkillers at $8.4 billion in 2011, and more than half the people who regularly take painkillers have back pain.

The cost of treating back pain appears to be higher in the United States than in most other developed countries. Our rate of back surgery, for example, is about twice the rate in Australia, New Zealand, most of Europe, and Canada. It's five times higher than in the United Kingdom. And Americans seem to have a unique conviction that high-tech treatments can solve all their medical problems.

Many people, perhaps most, assume that more medical care can only be better. Doctors are paid for doing more, not necessarily for doing better, so they're happy to deliver more care. That means more testing, more doctor visits, more surgery, and more drugs.

But are more of these things really better? This book considers what we know about treatments for back pain and asks a number of critical questions.

Are some of the most popular treatments really effective? Do they "cure" or even improve the problems they claim to address? If some back pain treatments are ineffective or even harmful, why do patients clamor for them and doctors provide them?

Who benefits from the vast back pain industry that's developed over the past thirty years? Is it patients? Or the doctors, hospitals, and manufacturers that produce the technology of back pain therapy?

What does all this say about our medical system? Or our efforts to enhance quality, improve safety, and reduce health care costs?

How can patients maneuver to help themselves rather than help the medical industry? Will efforts to measure patient satisfaction help deliver safer and more effective treatments or encourage the opposite?

In answering these questions, this book does more than describe and analyze the back business. It also explores the complex ways that doctors interact with patients, drug companies, and medical device makers. The results can inadvertently lead to treatments that are ineffective or even harmful.

These issues aren't unique to patients and doctors dealing with back pain. Back pain is a microcosm of broader problems in our health care system. As we'll see, well-meaning and popular solutions—often involving new drugs, devices, or even quality improvement efforts—may aggravate rather than solve the problems.

That's why so many people have a huge stake in understanding the back business. The first group of stakeholders is obviously back pain sufferers. If you have back pain, this book will help you take more control of the problem, avoid harm, and get your life back—or keep it.

Hope is an important part of getting better, and I want to convince you that even if there's not a definitive cure, your life is going to improve. Although you'll read here about many ineffective treatments, there are treatments that can help, and most require patients to take charge of their care.

So one goal of this book is to encourage more involvement in decisions about your own care. This doesn't mean insisting on a particular test or treatment against medical advice. It doesn't mean that medical advice is always wrong or that you can't trust your doctor. Rather, it means you need to become well informed and deeply involved in making decisions about your care. *Blindly* accepting professional recommendations—even though they're well meaning—may not always be a successful strategy.

David Freedman, a science and business journalist, wrote a book ominously titled *Wrong*. With many medical and business examples, he points out that a large fraction of expert advice is flawed. Regarding medical controversies, he remarks that humans "happen to be complex creatures living in a complex world, so why would we expect answers to *any* interesting question to be simple?"

He goes on to remind us that, given these complexities, any advice that's likely to be right is likely to be complex. It "will come with many qualifications. . . . Because of all the ifs, ands, or buts, it will be difficult to act on."

Even more frustrating, Freedman argues that we're all attracted to simple solutions and overly optimistic predictions. So genuinely good advice is often incompatible with our expectations. It's likely to be at odds with every aspect of the advice we *want* to believe.

What about the latest and greatest cures for back pain reported in the media? These cures appear on an almost daily basis. Freedman suggests being wary of advice that gets favorable attention from the press, the online crowd, or your friends. The problem is that the popularity of an idea is likely to reflect good promotion, provocativeness, or how well it resonates with the conventional wisdom rather than its likelihood of being right. We should beware of false messiahs.

I encourage avoiding a passive role not only in decision making but in physical activity. Don't treat back pain by going to bed rest, the standard treatment prescription when I was in medical training. Don't assume the cure will be found by lying in an MRI scanner. Don't assume it will be fixed by lying on an operating table. Don't assume that lying down for injections will be the cure. We'll see the fallacies in each of these assumptions.

In fact, resuming activities, increasing physical activity, and even vigorous exercise are often the keys to improving back pain—things no doctor or practitioner can do for you.

This leads to the second group of readers I hope to reach: the health care professionals who treat back pain. Although some may seem motivated by self-interest as much as by patient need, most are deeply caring and want to help.

That's one reason they continue to "do something," even when that something may not work. Doctors, physical therapists, and nurse practitioners, like so many Americans, have been socialized not to "just sit there" but to act.

The imperative to act is especially hard to resist when a suffering human being is sitting in your office begging for relief. Unfortunately, as we'll see, many of the things doctors recommend may be useless or worse. So providing those who treat back pain with a better understanding of the research evidence may help them do a better job with their patients.

Finally, I hope to reach policy makers and the media. The media have become an integral part of the medical industrial complex in general and the back business in particular. Miracle cures are a staple of popular health coverage. They attract an eager readership at magazine stands and bookstores and in cyberspace or the blogosphere.

There's nothing particularly sexy about exercise and yoga classes—activities that may be genuinely helpful for back pain. But the constant stream of "miracle cure" stories attracts hits. The problem is that it conveys a message to back pain sufferers that salvation lies in expensive treatments. Typically, treatments that are done to them rather than activities done by them.

If we want to deal effectively with back pain—not to mention our broader health care crisis—it's important that journalists, health reporters, and bloggers become more critical. They need to understand how to frame the issues, critically analyze the latest treatments, and translate this to a lay audience of patients and their families.

Policy makers also need to learn more about the genesis of the problems they're trying to solve. Back pain is a perfect policy laboratory. Our research into relationships between patients and doctors teaches us that putative silver bullets sometimes only make the problem worse. These silver bullets often include ever more intensive intervention, new technology, pain scales, and patient satisfaction questionnaires.

As we take a tour of the back business, many readers—particularly patients and doctors—may be deeply suspicious of my conclusions. Arguments to decrease use of specific medical services are often received with skepticism because this appears only to reduce quality of care and not improve it. Such a message will alarm readers who are convinced that certain treatments will work. As we'll see, even highly educated and influential people often insist on tests and treatments for back pain that are unlikely to help.

Other readers will question the motives of anyone who argues for less medical intervention, assuming that this reflects insensitivity to suffering, preoccupation with cost cutting, efforts to ration care, or a threat to patient autonomy. On the surface, cost containment seems to be the sole motivation. Insurance company maneuvers to limit their costs only reinforce these suspicions.

Glib pronouncements that "less is more" or that we're practicing "evidence-based medicine" are not reassuring. These phrases lead many people to conclude that something is being withheld—something that might have benefit. How could more testing and more information possibly be harmful? How could treatment that's more intensive possibly lead to worse results?

Answering these questions is part of the challenge of this book. A recurring theme is not to confuse doing more with doing what's best.

Have rapidly rising expenditures for back pain and a raft of new treatments helped? If more care and newer care were better, we might expect falling rates of activity limitation and work disability due to back pain. If all the surgical innovations of recent years were real improvements, we might see rates of *repeat* surgery going down. That is, we might expect that people would be doing so well after surgery, they wouldn't need more operations.

With heart disease, that seems to be just what's happening. Work disability from heart and blood vessel disease has been falling in recent decades. This is a result of better prevention and better treatment.

But for back pain, just the opposite is occurring. Annual surveys of people with back pain report steadily *worse* functional limitations over the past decade. Work disability due to back pain has been increasing. And rates of repeat surgery have been going up instead of down. This is both counterintuitive and emotionally unsatisfying.

But with back pain—as with many chronic diseases—there's a fundamental flaw in assuming that someone else is going to fix you. Nonetheless, they can get rich trying.

Let's be honest about a couple of things. First, research shows that most people with a recent onset of back pain—even severe back pain—will get better on their own, through natural healing processes. As a result, it's surprisingly hard to prove that treatments help in a new episode of back pain. That's because any treatment comparison has to beat this normal, rapid healing. Furthermore, because most people get better, it's easy to make the mistake of assuming that the improvement was the result of a particular treatment.

A fraction of people with back pain develop ongoing, unrelenting problems. Even more develop grumbling, low-level pain that flares up from time to time. For people with persistent or "chronic" pain, there are no magic bullets. I don't have a cure. To paraphrase a Frank Cotham cartoon in the *New Yorker*, I don't even have a race for the cure.

Most books and magazine articles on back pain offer *The Cure*. But notice . . . the cures are all different. And disabling back pain is increasing in the United States, despite the proliferation of cures.

The overabundance of cures, and variations in clinical practice from one doctor to the next, prompted my longtime colleague Dan Cherkin to subtitle an article we once wrote, "Who You See Is What

You Get." A New York pain specialist, Dr. Seth Waldman, put it slightly differently. "Each approach to diagnosis and treatment is essentially a franchise, and there are too many franchises battling for control."

Dr. Scott Haldeman is a medical neurologist *and* a chiropractor. As if that's not enough, he has a PhD in neurophysiology. His roots in South Africa are still audible when he speaks, and his education spans South Africa, Canada, and the United States. In a recent review, he and his colleagues counted more than two hundred available treatment options for chronic low back pain, without even considering surgery.

Now, if you have pernicious anemia, there's one treatment: vitamin B12. If you have thyroid deficiency, there's one treatment: thyroid hormone replacement. If you have appendicitis, there's generally one treatment: an appendectomy. But for back pain, there are more than two hundred options, plus dozens of different surgical procedures. If one treatment were overwhelmingly effective or clearly superior, this situation wouldn't exist.

Throughout this book, I'll be talking about lower back pain, which is more frequent than neck pain. And I'll be talking about the most common type of back pain—the type that's not caused by cancer, infection, or serious underlying disease. The type that's not associated with serious nerve injury that might cause foot or leg weakness, for example.

You may assume that you need an MRI to rule out these more serious conditions, but a careful office examination is usually all that's necessary. In fact, we'll look at some hazards of getting fancy tests when they aren't needed.

Overtesting and overtreatment turn out to be rampant in the back pain world. This partly explains why costs are skyrocketing while results are plunging. Again, this is hard to understand.

Hasn't medical research improved length and quality of life for people with AIDS? Isn't it true that kidney transplants do the same for people with end-stage kidney failure? Don't people with hip replacements get to play tennis again? Why aren't the results of care for back pain similarly improving?

Peter Pronovost is an intensive care doctor at Johns Hopkins Medical School in Baltimore. Clean-shaven and with a full head of light brown hair, he looks like a handsome athlete. He's famous for reducing complications in intensive care units by simply using checklists, as pilots do before flying, to avoid overlooking simple steps.

Pronovost argues that we have two American health care systems: "one that leads the world in discoveries and the other that often harms rather than heals." He also reminds us of consistent best estimates that the U.S. health care system wastes one-third of all spending—about $900 billion a year—on errors, waste, and inefficient care.

I argue that care for back pain is part of Pronovost's second health care system. Care for back pain is low-hanging fruit, where we could easily improve care and cut costs at the same time. In fact, it's the poster child for medical waste. Much of this is the result of an entire industry built around pain, taking advantage of vulnerable people who are often desperate for explanations and relief.

So over the next chapters we'll look closely at research on the efficacy of most popular back pain treatments. We'll examine what we know about them and then, at the end of the book, turn to what really works. In the course of this exploration, we'll learn why people may be "helped" by ineffective treatments, why doctors continue to prescribe them, and what we can do to break this cycle. I'll conclude with recommendations designed to promote better treatment, less pain and suffering, and lower health care costs.

I've had the opportunity to treat many patients with back pain and to conduct some key back pain research. Our studies have challenged and changed the standard of back care in the United States and around the world. Most of these studies have passed the test of time and helped patients and health care providers alike.

Yet even the best scientific studies draw opposition by threatening the status quo and the lucrative back pain industry. As a medical editor reminds us, once an industry builds up around an idea, research evidence gets politicized. Good research may get lost in a blizzard of opinion pieces.

So I've taken my share of flak at major spine conferences. This can happen when you challenge outmoded thinking and dare to suggest that some popular treatments aren't safe and effective. I quickly learned that dealing with disagreement and controversy is part and parcel of being a scientist. Let me offer some stories of my baptism in the back pain business and how I came to be convinced that some treatments are overused.

Going to Bed for Back Pain

When I started my medical career in the 1980s, the standard treatment for back pain was bed rest. Strict bed rest. You were not to get out of bed for meals. You were not to sit up in bed. We debated whether it was okay to go to the bathroom or whether a bedside commode was necessary. No one questioned the value of bed rest. We argued instead whether it had to be for two weeks or whether one week could suffice. But we prescribed some kind of bed rest for everyone with back pain.

Have you ever tried staying in bed for two weeks without sitting up? It's hard even to imagine. Even watching TV would require having it bolted to the ceiling. It was a prescription destined to drive people mad. And two weeks of bed rest is enough to cause muscle weakness and deconditioning of the heart and lungs. Fortunately, I doubt that anyone actually followed our instructions, and many admitted that they didn't.

We'd see those patients back in the office a few weeks later for follow-up. I'd often ask if they'd finished the bed rest as prescribed. The usual response was a chagrined, "Well, I tried it for a couple of days but really couldn't do it any longer than that." Or, "Well, I couldn't afford to miss work that long, so I had to cut it short."

"Well, is your back feeling better?" I'd ask. "Oh yeah, it's quite a bit better now" was the usual response.

Here was an odd disconnect. Most patients weren't following our instructions at all, but most were getting better anyway. What if the conventional wisdom was just wrong?

When I looked for scientific studies on the effectiveness of bed rest, I couldn't find any. This seemed to be a treatment based on theory, lore, and authoritarian pronouncement rather than actual data.

The theory was that lying down minimized pressure in the discs of the spine, the cushions between the vertebrae. And there was research using large-bore needles positioned in the disc and attached to pressure transducers showing that was true. But no one had proven that disc pressure was a key source of pain or that bed rest made pain get better faster.

The decision seemed to matter. Even though bed rest wasn't a treatment we billed for, the stakes for a patient were high. A week or two of work absenteeism had financial risks, and for some might even jeopardize the job. Physical deconditioning was inevitable. Being immobile thins bones, weakens muscles, and increases the risk of blood clots in the legs.

So in the 1980s, having just finished a research fellowship, I wanted to test whether bed rest actually made any difference. In the face of some skepticism and anxiety, my colleagues and I designed a study to test the theory.

We would take patients from a walk-in clinic with a complaint of back pain and—with their consent—randomly assign them to a full week of bed rest or just two days. We had to persuade the human research ethics committee that it was reasonable to withhold a full week of bed rest. That was the standard of care, after all. We chose two days of bed rest as a comparison strategy because it just seemed too radical to recommend none at all.

We recruited more than two hundred patients, most with back pain for less than a month. Then we followed them up over three months. We found no difference at all between the two-day strategy and the seven-day strategy in terms of pain relief or return to normal activities.

The only difference in the results was in work absenteeism. Those who spent two days in bed missed an average of three days of work, compared with six days for those assigned to a week in bed. In essence, by prescribing bed rest, we were prescribing work absenteeism without any medical benefit. Some people might not be able to return to physically demanding jobs after just two days, but they didn't need to stay in bed.

Since that time, nine more randomized trials have come to essentially the same conclusion. And of course, several of those studies tested a strategy of no bed rest at all. The results of these studies hint that staying out of bed isn't merely as good but might be *better* than resting in bed. And the lack of benefit for bed rest seems to be true for people with sciatica as well as back pain alone. That's the electric shock–like pain in the leg that some people with back pain get.

Happily, doctors no longer prescribe bed rest for back pain.

A few years after our study, one of my colleagues, a neurologist with a wry sense of humor, kidded me about the consequences. Tongue firmly in cheek, he reminded me that our research had eliminated one of doctors' favorite excuses. "If someone with back pain didn't get better," he said, "we could always ask, 'Well, did you stay at strict bed rest for a week?'" When the answer was inevitably "no," we could always say, "Well, no wonder you didn't get better! You didn't follow my instructions!"

Of course, he was describing a classic strategy of blaming the victim. We had a good laugh and were both pleased that clinical practice was evolving away from this approach.

When the *New England Journal of Medicine* published our bed rest study, it got some attention in the news media because back pain is so common. I got a few angry letters from patients who felt I was taking a valuable treatment away from them. One wished me a lifetime of agonizing chronic back pain as retribution. I also got a few indignant letters from neurosurgeons, who just *knew* bed rest was critical and that patients would be harmed without it.

But overall, doctors accepted the study, and there was only modest controversy. I got invitations to lecture about the results, and they seemed to fit well with a growing sense that bed rest wasn't much use for this condition, or for anything else. No one was making money off bed rest, there was no market for bed rest, there was no industry supported by bed rest. It was an easy sell. Practice changed.

Contrast that with the impact of our next major research effort.

Less than Electrifying Results

Our next project was a study of transcutaneous electrical nerve stimulation, or TENS. TENS is a treatment that delivers mild electrical stimulation through several electrodes stuck to the skin. The stimulation comes from a device about the size of a deck of cards, which attaches easily to a belt and has wires to the electrodes.

Doctors also based this treatment on a theory—that sensation from an outside source could compete with pain signals to the brain, reducing the pain sensation. There was an analogy to rubbing your funny bone when you smack your elbow.

Companies initially developed TENS units as a way to screen for patients who might benefit from surgically implanted electrodes right next to the spinal cord. When some patients seemed to improve with a TENS unit alone, it became a treatment in its own right. But there was little rigorous proof that it worked.

So—again with patient consent—we assigned patients with persistent back pain to get a real TENS unit or a sham TENS unit. The sham units were identical to the real thing, with a flashing "on" light, but they delivered no electrical current.

Patients in both the true TENS and the sham TENS groups improved. In fact, both groups improved the same amount, at the same pace. The benefit of TENS appeared to be mostly a placebo effect.

The *New England Journal of Medicine* also published this study, and it got a lot of attention. This time, the response was more heated.

I found myself debating with the president of a TENS manufacturer on public radio. The company president argued that without the wonders of TENS, patients would be "condemned to the living hell of narcotic addiction," as if TENS or narcotics were the only treatment choices for back pain. Remember, Scott Haldeman identified two hundred different treatments for back pain described in the medical literature.

I found myself responding to angry letters from physical therapists, who often recommend and manage TENS therapy. Letters to the editors of clinical journals and newsletters attacked our study for years—and still do even today. It apparently hit a nerve that our study of bed rest didn't.

Sales of TENS units dipped for a while but then recovered. Nonetheless, a recent review of research studies (almost twenty years later) supported our results. It concluded that the highest-quality trials do "not support the use of TENS in the routine management of chronic low back pain." It also encouraged further research, because there are still few high-quality studies. Guidelines from the American Academy of Neurology similarly concluded, "TENS is not recommended for the treatment of chronic low back pain."

In 2012 the controversy led Medicare to encourage research that's more definitive. Medicare officials have taken the stance that they'll pay for TENS therapy only if patients agree to participate in such a study. The results may determine whether Medicare will continue insurance coverage for TENS.

This was my introduction to the influence of entrenched interests in managing back pain. The device manufacturers and therapists who favored TENS therapy had a major investment in the treatment. They vigorously resisted any suggestion that it might be no more than a placebo.

Unfortunately, their response was not to fund more and better research. Once a treatment has approval of the Food and Drug Administration (FDA), manufacturers have little to gain by doing more research.

You may assume that FDA approval of TENS units means they've been well tested and proven effective. But TENS units were introduced shortly before the FDA acquired authority over medical devices in 1976. At that time, devices already on the market were "grandfathered in" for approval. Furthermore, the FDA's early evaluation of medical devices focused on safety more than efficacy. And newer devices are widely approved on the basis of "substantial equivalence" to devices marketed before 1976.

I was beginning to learn about the back business. It's a for-profit business dedicated to selling products and generating return for stockholders.

Any benefit for patients is welcome but secondary. And as we'll see, the market comes close to including every American adult. It's a business that always assumes newer and more is better, despite growing evidence to the contrary. My immersion in the back Business had begun, but it was far from complete.

Fusing Spines

My real baptism came with research on spinal fusion surgery. This is an operation designed to join two vertebrae with bone grafts, an operation we'll discuss later in more detail. It's most often performed today with screws inserted into the vertebrae, and connecting rods or plates to immobilize the vertebrae while the bone grafts heal. This hardware is expensive and profitable, adding thousands of dollars to the cost of a single back operation. The most popular gadgets are called pedicle screws, which were relatively new at the time we naively embarked on a new research project.

As the TENS project was being published, our research team received funding from the federal Agency for Health Care Policy and Research. Congress gave this new agency responsibility for improving the effectiveness and efficiency of health care rather than making laboratory discoveries.

One part of our research focused on spinal fusion surgery. Our critical review of the available research suggested that there were few scientifically validated indications for this type of surgery. Our research also suggested that this type of surgery resulted in greater costs and complications than simpler forms of back surgery.

At the same time, the agency sponsored a guideline panel to summarize the research literature on back pain, and I was a member of the panel. The chair was an orthopedic surgeon, and the panel included three other orthopedic and neurosurgeons. The entire panel had twenty-three members, representing nearly every profession and specialty with an interest in back pain. The panel limited itself to back pain of recent onset, or "acute" low back pain, and concluded that nonsurgical treatments were most often appropriate. Regarding fusion surgery, all the studies we found addressed persistent back pain, so there was no evidence that it helped for acute pain.

The research and guideline efforts were simply too much for the North American Spine Society, a group made up mainly of spine surgeons. The society had close ties to the companies that make screws and rods for fusion surgery. The Spine Society argued that our research and the guidelines were biased against their preferred forms of therapy. The group inspired a letter-writing campaign to Congress, and some members formed a lobbying group with the stated goal of eliminating the funding agency.

One screw manufacturer, AcroMed, sought a subpoena of all our research records and communications at the University of Washington. Another company, Sofamor Danek, sought a court injunction to block release of the back pain guidelines. Neither effort was successful, but they exposed the role of device manufacturers in opposing our research and the production of guidelines.

The Agency for Health Care Policy and Research became a political target not only because of lobbying related to back pain but also because a new Congress was eager to cut government spending as part of its "Contract with America." Further, Republican members of Congress saw the agency and its new head as advocates for the Clinton health plan, which they opposed.

In one budget draft, the House of Representatives eliminated the agency. However, many medical groups and hospital organizations came to the support of the agency, and it survived with endorsement of the Senate—but with a 25 percent budget cut. Political pressure related to the back pain guidelines led the agency to stop sponsoring the production of guidelines, despite a congressional mandate when the agency was established. And despite the fact that guidelines could be useful to thousands or even millions of patients and their doctors.

The North American Spine Society later faced allegations that some of its continuing medical education programs were thinly disguised promotions for the spinal screws. The plaintiffs, patients alleging bad results from pedicle screws, likened the educational seminars to Tupperware parties.

Courts dismissed suits against the Spine Society for lack of evidence, but suits against the device manufacturers went forward. AcroMed, which had subpoenaed our research records, settled thousands of patient lawsuits alleging bad results, for $100 million. The company did not acknowledge any liability.

Years later, in 2006, Sofamor Danek's parent company, Medtronic, reached a $40 million settlement with the federal government over allegations of kickbacks to spine surgeons. The company denied any wrongdoing, but the Justice Department described the kickbacks as "sham consulting agreements, sham royalty agreements and lavish trips."

Also in 2006, the successor to the Agency for Health Care Policy and Research (the Agency for Healthcare Research and Quality, or AHRQ) sponsored a systematic review of the research literature on use of spine fusion surgery for a common diagnosis, degeneration of spinal discs. By that time, there were some strong research studies, all from Europe, that we hadn't had in the mid-1990s. That draft review concluded, "Fusion for degenerative disc disease has no conclusive advantage over nonsurgical treatment, either in the short-term or the long-term."

Despite research findings and allegations against the manufacturers, sales of pedicle screws and similar spinal devices have risen steadily since our research in the 1990s, thanks in part to aggressive marketing. According to government statistics, spinal fusion surgery of all sorts increased 660 percent between 1993 and 2010. The proportion of operations involving pedicle screws or similar hardware has increased as well, so that surgeons now use these devices in the vast majority of fusion operations.

Even some surgeons find the increase alarming. Dr. Edward Benzel, a neurosurgeon at the prestigious Cleveland Clinic, estimated that fewer than half the spinal fusions being performed were appropriate.

"The reality of it is, we all cave in to market and economic forces," he told the *New York Times* in 2003. In the same article, Yale University neurosurgeon Zoher Ghogawala added, "I see too many patients who are recommended a fusion that absolutely do not need it."

The *Times* also quoted Stan Mendenhall, the editor and publisher of *Orthopedic Network News*. Mendenhall said, "A lot of technological innovation serves shareholders more than patients. . . . The money is driving a lot of this." And spine fusion rates have continued to climb steeply since those comments a decade ago.

We might note that none of these investigations has prompted Congress to substantially expand AHRQ's budget or restore its mandate to sponsor development of clinical guidelines.

In retrospect, each of our research projects inflamed opponents who had strong beliefs or market share in a particular approach to back pain. None welcomed evidence that conflicted with strongly held opinions. And some were big businesses that seemed eager to avoid scrutiny of their products while profiting from patients with back pain. These experiences became the germ of my conviction that we're overusing many treatments for back pain.

What's the real evidence that some treatments for back pain are overused? Does research support this conclusion? This book addresses these questions and many more. It's the first comprehensive look into what has become a vast and lucrative industry purporting to address back pain, a problem that afflicts millions of Americans.

As we look for more evidence of overuse, I'll introduce a number of back pain sufferers, some of them quite famous. You may figure that you're smart enough to avoid the pitfalls. But even the best and brightest among us have sometimes stumbled when it comes to getting treated for back pain. We'll take a look at some of these individuals over the course of this book and see what we can learn from their experiences.

Chapter 2

EVEN THE BEST
AND BRIGHTEST

We know a lot about managing back pain, but many patients never get adequate care. Even celebrities and those in prominent positions sometimes encounter quicksand when they seek care for back pain.

David Fridovich is a tough guy. He was a star linebacker in college, then a Green Beret. In fact, he became a three-star general and deputy commander of the nation's elite Special Forces—the Green Berets, Army Rangers, Navy SEALS, and Delta Force.

Cindy McCain is a savvy businesswoman and philanthropist. She chaired one of the largest beer distributors in the United States, became the wife of Senator John McCain, and adopted an orphan from Bangladesh. She took up racecar driving and flying in her spare time.

Jerome Groopman is a famous doctor and author. He's a professor of medicine at Harvard Medical School and a leading researcher in cancer and AIDS. In all his spare time, he pens articles for the *New Yorker* and writes best-selling books.

John F. Kennedy was the king of Camelot. He served all too briefly as the thirty-fifth president of the United States.

What do these four have in common, other than being smart, ambitious, talented, and successful? Like most of us at some time, they were plagued by back pain. *Unlike* many of us, by virtue of position or wealth, they had access to the best health care in the world. And yet, to make matters worse, all suffered at the hands of medical professionals they consulted.

Consider the experience of President Kennedy. What he thought was the best medical care in the world bought him two failed back operations, life-threatening complications, a raft of fruitless injections, a useless corset, and years of unnecessary pain. He improved only after pursuing a rigorous exercise program created by Dr. Hans Kraus, a pioneer of sports medicine.

Like Kennedy, the others found benefits from proven low-tech treatments after suffering through unproven high-tech treatments. We shouldn't conclude that all novel or high-tech back pain treatments are useless—but many are overused.

Kennedy's instructive medical history illustrates many of the themes of this book. So let's take a closer look at the history of his back pain and the mistakes he and his doctors made. Then we'll consider the lessons that modern patients can glean from his experiences. Even though his story is decades old, and treatments have ostensibly advanced since the 1960s, many modern patients have similar experiences. In fact, you may conclude that little has changed.

We now have details of Kennedy's back problems, thanks to recent work by both historians and doctors. The relevant medical records became accessible only in 2002 because they had been guarded by friends of the Kennedy administration. Most recently, the family of Dr. Hans Kraus donated some of Kennedy's private medical records to the Kennedy Presidential Library in 2006, filling in events from Kennedy's final years. I had a chance to review Kraus's records at the Kennedy Library.

A Presidential Problem

According to military records, Kennedy began having "an occasional pain in his right sacro-iliac joint" as early as age twenty-one. Kennedy himself described sudden back pain after a tennis match during college, reporting that it felt like "something had slipped." His mother, Rose Kennedy, cited a football injury as yet another possible cause of Kennedy's back pain.

With the outbreak of World War II, Kennedy tried to volunteer for both the Army and the Navy, but both rejected him because of back problems. At that point, Kennedy undertook a personal exercise program. A subsequent medical examination in 1941 deemed him fit for duty, though Kennedy sought further evaluation of his back problems shortly thereafter.

A Boston doctor judged that Kennedy did not have a herniated disc, often called a "slipped disc." The doctor wrote, "I don't think this is a disc since the pain . . . does not even remotely resemble a disc—no interference with reflexes, nothing pointing to a spinal condition."

A Navy neurosurgeon agreed that Kennedy's pain wasn't consistent with sciatica. Sciatica is the electric shock of pain and tingling that travel down the leg when a herniated disc pinches a spinal nerve. His doctors recommended against surgery.

Kennedy was working in the Secretary of the Navy's office when the Japanese attacked Pearl Harbor, but he wanted a combat assignment. After training, he took command of a patrol torpedo (PT) boat in the Pacific.

Kennedy's crew members were aware of his ongoing back problems. He slept with a plywood board under his mattress and wore a "corset-type thing." A colleague wrote that Kennedy refused to report to sick bay and "feigned being *well.*"

During a nighttime patrol in the Solomon Islands, in pitch-black conditions, a Japanese destroyer rammed Kennedy's PT 109. Kennedy was at the wheel, but the impact threw him against the rear wall of the boat's cockpit, where his back slammed against a steel reinforcing brace.

Military records documented Kennedy's subsequent heroics. Despite his reinjured back, Kennedy towed a badly burned crewman three miles through open ocean with a life-jacket strap clenched in his teeth. This and other actions won Kennedy the Navy and Marine Corps Medal.

But the war took a toll on Kennedy's back problems, which worsened after the sinking of PT 109. It remains unclear if this was a result of the collision, the strenuous rescue effort, or simply the worsening of an ongoing condition.

After Kennedy returned to the United States, doctors reevaluated him for back surgery. Though still in the Navy, in 1944 Kennedy went to the New England Baptist Hospital with his family's financial support. Here neurosurgeon James Poppen operated on Kennedy for a presumed herniated disc. Following surgery, though, Poppen wrote, "There, however, was very little protrusion of the ruptured cartilage."

Ordinarily, successful disc surgery results in prompt relief. Instead, Kennedy had persistent pain, a prolonged hospitalization, and a resulting transfer to the Chelsea Naval Hospital. Poppen attributed the ongoing pain to severe muscle spasms.

At the naval hospital, the neurosurgeon who had seen Kennedy before deployment to the Solomon Islands reassessed the situation. He questioned the need for surgery. While in the hospital, Kennedy wrote to a girlfriend, saying, "In regard to the fascinating subject of my operation I . . . think the doc should have read just one more book before picking up the saw."

After reviewing the records, my orthopedist colleague Robert Hart said of the surgery, "It was probably a misdiagnosis, but the surgeon in that case did what any surgeon would do—he went ahead and removed the disk anyway." Hart also noted that X-rays a few months after surgery were normal, with no signs of wear in the discs or vertebrae and nothing that would make the spine unstable.

Kennedy was from a political family, so it was no surprise that after his Navy discharge, he ran for Congress. He had persistent back problems through a vigorous political campaign. Those close to him described frequent use of steaming hot tub baths and a lumbar corset. The campaign was successful despite the back problems. Kennedy won by a wide margin and served in Congress for six years.

In 1952, Kennedy moved into the Senate after defeating incumbent Republican Henry Cabot Lodge Jr. While campaigning, he often walked with crutches to relieve his spine. During his first Senate term, Kennedy's back pain progressed, and he became unbearable to work with. His personal secretary of twelve years, Evelyn Lincoln, wrote that she considered finding a new job.

By 1954, X-rays showed that the disc space where Kennedy had surgery had completely collapsed, leaving essentially no cushion between the adjacent vertebrae. Some early bone spurs were beginning to form. My colleague, Bob Hart, reviewed the X-rays and found no sign of osteoporosis or vertebral compression fractures, contradicting some historians.

That year, at age thirty-seven, Kennedy discussed further back surgery at New York's Hospital for Special Surgery. Despite increased risks due to other medical problems, Kennedy and his doctors decided to proceed with a spinal fusion operation at the site of the previous disc surgery. Doctors told Kennedy that a fusion procedure would strengthen his lower spine and that without it he might lose his ability to walk.

His father, Joe Kennedy, tried to dissuade Kennedy from surgery. But Rose Kennedy later said, "Jack was determined to have the operation. He told his father that even if the risks were fifty-fifty, he would rather be dead than spend the rest of his life hobbling on crutches and paralyzed by pain."

Kennedy underwent the spinal fusion procedure, an operation that welds vertebrae together with bone grafts. The operation included placement of a metal implant made of cobalt-chromium. Such implanted plates were relatively new: a high-tech aspect of Kennedy's treatment.

The postoperative course went poorly. Perhaps because of a serious urinary infection, Kennedy at one point lapsed into unconsciousness, and a priest performed last rites. When he finally left the hospital, Kennedy went to recover at a family home in Palm Beach, Florida.

But an infection brewed at the site of his surgery. In 1955, he returned to the hospital for his third spine operation: to remove the metal plates and surgically clean the infected wound.

While recovering from this operation, Kennedy consulted with Dr. Janet Travell. Travell, a specialist in internal medicine and pain medicine, eventually became his personal doctor. Asked about the cause of Kennedy's back pain, Travell found it impossible "to reconstruct by hindsight what might have happened to him over the years." However, in her opinion, Kennedy "resented" the back operations, which "seemed to only make him worse."

Travell later recommended a rocking chair for Kennedy, believing it helped his back. She also began trigger point injections with procaine, a local anesthetic. Kennedy's diagnosis when he left the hospital was sacroiliac and lumbar pain with continued muscle spasm.

In 1957, Dr. Travell diagnosed a recurrent abscess of the lumbar spine and admitted Kennedy once again to the Hospital for Special Surgery. In Kennedy's fourth spine operation, surgeons drained a staph abscess and removed dead tissue.

In 1960, Kennedy mounted his successful campaign for the presidency. At that point, he was determined to present the picture of health and vigor, declaring himself in "excellent" shape. But in the White House, Kennedy received regular medical care from a phalanx of doctors, among them Travell, Admiral George Burkley, and a doctor who had immigrated from Germany, Max Jacobson. Jacobson had the reputation for treating celebrities with "pep pills" (amphetamines), and patients nicknamed him "Dr. Feelgood."

Jacobson treated Kennedy with injections of a bizarre cocktail of vitamins, hormones, amphetamines, and other ingredients. Kennedy thought these made him less dependent on crutches and once dismissed questions about the injections by saying, "I don't care if it's horse piss. It works."

However, Burkley concluded in 1961 that Kennedy's various passive treatments, including injections, back braces, ultrasound, and hot packs, were doing more harm than good. He observed what Kennedy tried to hide from the press: that the president went up and down helicopter stairs one at a time, rose only with difficulty from sitting, and often relied on crutches. Fearing the president might end up in a wheelchair, he pressed Travell to consult Dr. Hans Kraus.

Kraus was an Austrian immigrant who specialized in rehabilitation medicine. He was an exercise advocate and had worked with President Eisenhower to establish the President's Council on Physical Fitness. A mountaineer and rock climber who married a downhill ski champion, Kraus was well known to athletes. Some describe him as the father of sports medicine in the United States.

A biographer noted, "Dr. Kraus's approach was controversial within the American medical establishment. He relied strongly on strengthening and stretching exercises, common sense, and avoiding surgery at all costs. His treatments were seemingly old-fashioned, time-consuming and relatively unprofitable for a doctor." Nonetheless, he had a celebrity clientele that included Katharine Hepburn, Eleanor Roosevelt, Yul Brynner, and Angela Lansbury.

Records in the Kennedy Library show that Kraus examined JFK in October 1961 and concluded, "Weakness and stiffness of key posture muscles may well account for some of the persistent pain and acute episodes. . . . We should try a program of gradually increasing strengthening exercises for weak muscles, and limbering and stretching exercises for stiff muscles. . . . I would be in favor of injecting as little as possible."

Kennedy began to exercise three times a week in a small White House gym. He followed a regimen of aerobics, strengthening, and flexibility exercises, all to the strains of his favorite country-and-western and show tunes.

Along with massage and heat therapy, this regimen became a respite for Kennedy from his busy schedule. Nonetheless, Kraus's notes repeatedly indicate that, given competing demands, Kennedy was not as adherent to the program as Kraus would have liked.

Even so, the exercise program produced results within weeks. A *New York Times* article in December 1961 noted, "President Kennedy still is swimming and taking muscle-strengthening exercises every day. . . . His bad back apparently is tremendously better. . . . Dr. Kraus still makes the visit once or twice a week, Presidential aides said, and he has done wonders for the President."

Later press reports were even more admiring. In July 1962, a White House correspondent wrote, "Getting on and off his Air Force jet, Mr. Kennedy no longer walks up and down the ramp with the cautious air of a man waiting for something to snap. . . . Memories are short, but last June the President was hobbling on crutches, being lifted into his aircraft by a crane. . . . Mr. Kennedy has not used the crutches again, his associates say, and has not been seriously troubled by his back since a siege at Christmastime in Palm Beach."

Kennedy continued exercise for the remainder of his life. His doctors reduced the injections. Kraus was convinced that Kennedy's corset was more hindrance than help and planned to wean Kennedy from it. But the assassination—in November 1963—prevented that milestone.

Following Kennedy's assassination, Admiral Burkley wrote to thank Kraus: "You returned the President to a full life allowing him to enjoy the activities and sports he so dearly loved."

Evelyn Lincoln, Kennedy's long-time assistant, wrote to Kraus years later. She declared, "I was in a position to know which doctors helped him. . . . I had full confidence in you, and I wasn't disappointed. From the very beginning, I could notice increasing mobility and as the treatment progressed he was becoming a man with 'vigah.' I have often stated that in the last six months . . . he was in the best health he had ever been. And a thing he was able to do, was to pick little John up and toss him around—something that had been lacking in his life."

Lessons from a President's Back Pain

JFK suffered a lifetime of maddening back pain. But his experience offers several lessons, each of which we'll elaborate in later chapters.

Let's start with the initial cause of his back pain. Was it a tennis match, a football injury, or something else? Many people with back pain—perhaps most—can't confidently name an inciting event when the pain began. Often the onset is insidious. Many ascribe chronic back pain to an "injury," but injured tissues heal in a matter of months, not a lifetime. Like headaches, which we usually don't ascribe to injury, backaches often have little to do with trauma.

Furthermore, most of us have back pain as an adult, even without football, combat injuries, or jobs involving heavy lifting. Indeed, a sedentary lifestyle may be a risk factor. Back pain is a predictable part of life, though we're just getting glimmers of why it's so persistent for some people.

Kennedy tried a wide range of treatments, from corsets to surgery, pills to injections, ultrasound to massage, hot packs to exercise. A plethora of treatments and specialists promise cures for back pain. Where many treatments exist, you can bet that the cause of the problem is elusive and that none of the treatments is uniquely effective.

Kennedy's surgery suggests the cliché that if you have a hammer, everything looks like a nail. Specialists trained in a narrow expertise tend to see their pet conditions, and apply pet therapies, in nearly every situation. How else do we explain that Kennedy got surgery for a herniated disc when there was little to suggest that was the problem? As my colleague Bob Hart said, his surgeon "did what any surgeon would do—he went ahead and removed the disk anyway."

It's unwise to pursue surgery just because nothing else has worked. Indeed, failure of previous treatment isn't an indication for spine surgery. Surgery aims at correcting specific anatomical abnormalities. If there's not a clear and correctible anatomical cause of the symptoms— or if an irrelevant anatomical abnormality gets fixed—surgery won't relieve the pain. Kennedy learned that the hard way with two operations, despite his conviction that surgery would help.

Kennedy's second back operation was a spine fusion with metal implants. As we'll see, this type of treatment has exploded in popularity among surgeons, even though there's considerable controversy about when it's actually effective. In Kennedy's case, it didn't help, and he suffered serious complications. Postoperative infections remain a concern even today. Doctors and patients alike tend to underestimate the risks of many medical and surgical treatments.

What worked for Kennedy? When he wanted to pass his military physical, it was exercise. After failed back surgery and injections, it was exercise. Passively being operated on, injected, medicated, and corseted didn't work. Exercise relieved much of Kennedy's pain, returned him to recreational sports, and let him toss his young son. It restored much of his quality of life. His challenge, as for most of us, was sticking with an exercise program in the face of a busy life.

So another important theme, supported today by better scientific evidence, is that active self-care, physical activity, and regular exercise are key features of treatment for chronic back pain. High-tech therapy and having things done *to* him were not the keys to success for JFK.

Kennedy continued to have recurrences of back pain, and exercise wasn't a "cure" in the usual sense. But the exercise made a huge difference in his quality of life. Though some doctors and marketing messages imply that we can always cure pain, it's simply not true—even with the best medical care. It wasn't true in the 1960s, nor is it today. But that doesn't mean pain can't be treated.

Ambiguous onset, diagnostic uncertainty, multiple treatments with modest efficacy, specialists pursuing pet treatments, and ultimately the importance of active self-care: these remain pervasive themes in the back pain world. For Kennedy, focusing on daily function proved more helpful than focusing on pain alone.

Kennedy's story reminds us that even severe back problems need not prevent a high-level career and active life. Fortunately, Kennedy didn't have to lift crates or work on an assembly line. But he was in perhaps the most stressful job in the world (the Cuban missile crisis comes to mind), engaged in frequent national and international travel, and was constantly in the public spotlight. By any definition, Kennedy had chronic pain, but he coped with it amazingly well.

Kennedy's experience suggests that making better-informed decisions, pursuing good self-care, and choosing active rather than passive treatment approaches go farther than expecting "magic bullets." We'll take a look at others who, like JFK, learned this the hard way.

When all was said and done, what was Kennedy's diagnosis? Muscle spasm? Herniated disc? Sacroiliac joint pain? Weakness and stiffness of posture muscles? Various doctors at various times made all these diagnoses, even before the complications of surgery and spinal abscesses. Historians have assigned diagnoses of congenitally unstable spine, vertebral compression fractures, and osteoporosis, but there's nothing to support these claims. His X-rays were normal up to the time he had disc surgery and shortly thereafter.

Diagnostic uncertainty is the norm in back care, though doctors hate to admit it. In spite of back pain since his college years, there was nothing on Kennedy's X-rays to show a cause of pain. Indeed, imaging tests don't show pain. Many patients believe that if imaging tests are normal, doctors must think the pain is "all in their heads." But Kennedy's example is more the rule than the exception, and no one thought he was malingering. Remember—he feigned being *well*.

Even with modern tests like magnetic resonance imaging (MRI) scans, the correct diagnosis is usually frustratingly elusive. Newer imaging tests have in some ways aggravated the problem—by revealing spine abnormalities even in people who *don't* have pain. This makes it hard to distinguish relevant from irrelevant findings. While we can sometimes affix a clear diagnosis, pinpointing a precise anatomical cause is impossible most of the time.

Modern imaging creates the illusion that we can always identify the cause of back pain and therefore always pick the right treatment. How could that not be true?

Chapter 3

WHAT'S WRONG?
WHAT'S NOT? CAN WE
TELL THE DIFFERENCE?

Seeing is believing. And seeing inside the body is an irresistible chance to discover what's wrong. A blood sugar is an abstract notion to most of us. So is a bone density score, a cholesterol level, or even a blood pressure.

But a bulging disc! Thanks to the miracles of modern imaging, like the MRI, we can take a picture and *see* that! Furthermore, knowing about a bulging disc can only be good, right? Knowledge is power. More information can only be better, and information seems harmless. And with an MRI, there's not even radiation exposure!

Most of us are uncomfortable with uncertainty, especially when it comes to our health. We often request tests to reduce that anxiety, and our family members may feel guilty if they don't press for every test that might help. An extra test, "just to be sure," seems preferable to missing something. People in pain may be especially eager for active testing and treatment, even if some of the options are unlikely to help. "Don't just stand there—do something!" is how most of us feel when we're in pain.

So why do the clinical guidelines from eleven countries—including the United States—recommend against doing X-rays for the vast majority of people with recent onset of back pain? And why do U.S. guidelines recommend doing MRI or CT (computed tomography) scans for only the unusual patient with extenuating circumstances? Is it just to save money?

Before we get into the research on MRI scans, it helps to review a little spinal anatomy. Remember that the spine consists of a series of stacked bones, the vertebrae, separated by cushions called discs. The discs not only provide cushioning; they allow the movement that enables a golf swing or picking up a baby.

Those discs are made of cartilage, but they're built a little like a jelly donut—maybe a stale jelly donut. That is, they have a tough outer rim and softer material in the center. If the tough rim develops cracks, as it always does with aging, the softer material inside can squeeze out, and that's what we call a herniated disc. If you're unlucky, that squeezed material may pinch a nerve that comes from the spinal cord. That can cause the "electric shock" type of pain in the leg and foot that we call sciatica.

But remember that there are lots of things in the spine that can cause pain besides discs pinching nerves. The vertebrae also have small joints that articulate between them, called facet joints. Although they're small, these joints get arthritis just like knees, hips, and other joints. This can result from wear on the cartilage of the joint and inflammation. The bones themselves have nerves and can cause pain, as in a fracture.

And those vertebrae aren't just loosely stacked, like blocks in a kid's playroom. A tough casing of ligaments and muscles surrounds them and attaches to them, providing stability while allowing movement. It's as if they're shrink-wrapped but with flexible material. And those ligaments and muscles can be painful, just like ligaments and muscles anywhere in the body. The point is that it can be darned tricky in an individual person to figure out where the pain is coming from.

Imaging tests like MRI scans produce astonishing pictures of the inside of the body. Even doctors are still amazed at what we can see. But imaging tests show anatomy, and not pain. And there's a growing problem with our sophisticated imaging: it's so detailed that it uncovers anatomical things that have nothing to do with a patient's symptoms. That creates the possibility of red herrings. We think we know what's causing the symptoms, when we really don't. And those red herrings can lead to unnecessary additional tests and treatments.

This isn't just a problem in the spine. Glands like the adrenal gland and the pituitary gland can show nodules on MRI that we just don't know how to interpret. Most often, they have no clinical importance at all. In this sense, they're just incidental findings, and doctors have adopted the tongue-in-cheek term "incidentalomas" to describe them.

How do we know there can be red herrings in the spine? Because people who have no back pain at all can have horrible-looking spines on MRI scans. Dr. Scott Boden was among the first to demonstrate this problem.

Boden is a wiry and intense orthopedic surgeon at Emory University in Atlanta who specializes in spine surgery. He's had a long career of award-winning research and patient care. He's also the proud father of amazingly accomplished triplet girls, and a serious baseball fan. On the research side, one of his major interests is spine imaging.

Dr. Boden managed to find sixty-seven adults who claimed, at least, that they had never had back pain or sciatica. They ranged from twenty to eighty years old. These people all agreed to have MRI scans, and three expert radiologists—the people who read scans and X-rays—interpreted the pictures independently. Among these sixty-seven "normal" people, one-quarter had a herniated disc, sometimes also called a "slipped disc."

If a herniated disc doesn't pinch a nerve, it may cause no pain at all. Even if it comes in contact with a nerve, there may be little pain if the pressure is not too great and if there's not much inflammation. Inflammation refers to redness, swelling, and heat that can affect the nerve and cause pain. So the people in Boden's study had no back pain and no leg pain but a herniated disc on MRI nonetheless. You can imagine that if you and your doctor discovered a herniated disc, you'd think you knew the cause of any back pain. But it might be a red herring, as it apparently was in these people.

And that's not all. Most of the normal people in this study—60 percent—had a bulging disc. That's a disc that bulges a little beyond its usual boundaries, but the soft interior hasn't squeezed out. So a bulging disc is normal. In fact, that's what discs are supposed to do as they provide cushioning. Normal means they bulge a little here and there with stress and pressure but don't break.

Looking further, more than half these normal people had degenerated discs. That term sounds awful. I've had patients describe that condition back to me as a "dissolving spine." Doctors have probably caused some harm just frightening people with that label.

But a degenerative disc is simply one of the earliest signs of aging. It's like gray hair and wrinkles but often happens even sooner. A third of the normal people under age forty had degenerative discs in Boden's study. It means the disc is losing some of its normal water content and may be getting thinner, but it doesn't mean there's anything wrong.

Boden's study found that among people over age sixty, all these findings were even more common. In that age group, the vast majority had a bulging disc, and all but one person had degenerated discs. On average, each person had three degenerated discs! So it would be more abnormal *not* to have these findings over age sixty than to have them. A variety of other MRI abnormalities is also common in normal people without back pain.

Why do some people get degenerated discs at an early age? If you're one of the unlucky ones with bad-looking discs under age forty, is it because of something you did? Sports? Strenuous work? Too much gardening? Probably not.

Studies of twins suggest this is mostly a result of genetics, just like gray hair. That is to say, identical twins have very similar-looking spines, even if they've pursued very different life paths with very different demands on their spines. One study found the MRIs nearly identical when one twin was a computer programmer and the other a plumber. Or when one was a journalist and the other a farmer. So our spines all change with age, but the pace may be predetermined.

Now suppose you're a skeptic, as you should be. You might reasonably ask, what if the sixty-seven people Boden recruited were a little unusual and not typical of normal people? After all, sixty-seven is a pretty small sample. But this study has been replicated about a dozen times. And the percentage of "abnormal" findings in "normal" people is pretty consistent. This seems to be the true state of affairs.

You might also ask, what about CT scans or other imaging tests? The same problems occur, and the frequency of abnormal findings is strikingly similar.

And another question may pop into your head. What happens to these people over time? Don't the MRI findings just get worse? Don't these abnormalities just predict problems down the road, even if they're not a problem now?

It's true that degenerative changes gradually increase as we get older, as Boden's study suggests. But that's just part of aging. If we look at herniated discs, it turns out that the imaging picture usually improves over time, in a matter of months. The herniated part of the disc seems to shrink in a natural healing process. That may be why most people with a herniated disc gradually get better even without surgery. More about that in a later chapter.

The same thing is true for bulging discs. Many just get better over time.

My colleague Dr. Jerry Jarvik is a neuroradiologist at the University of Washington, someone who specializes in reading images of the brain and spinal cord. He comes from a family of famous doctors and medical researchers, and his major research interest is back pain. He's thin, with a head of unruly, curly brown hair. He manages to be both energetic and thoughtful of those around him, and is quite willing to challenge the conventional wisdom.

Dr. Jarvik led our Seattle research team in a study similar to Boden's, in which he collected a group of people without back pain, did MRI scans, and then followed up on them three years later. At the outset, their frequency of "abnormalities" was much like that among Boden's subjects.

Sure enough, at follow-up, two-thirds of those people had developed back pain. Remember I said nearly everyone would have it sooner or later. But the striking thing was that the initial MRI was a bad predictor of who would get back pain over those three years. And there were very few new abnormalities that cropped up on the repeat MRI scans. It turned out that a diagnosis of depression at the beginning of the study was a stronger predictor of who would get back pain than the MRI results were.

That's not to say that back pain is simply a result of a bad mood or that it's all in your head. More on that later, too. It's just to say that anatomic changes on a scan may be only weakly related to pain symptoms.

But here's the problem. Once you know you have a bulging disc, or a herniated disc, or a degenerated disc, you can't get it out of your mind. It may have nothing to do with your pain. Your doctor may reassure you on that score—although many don't. But there's always a nagging question in the back of your mind. Could this be causing my pain? Am I going to make it worse if I run, or play golf, or pick up the baby? Shouldn't I get that fixed?

It may sound far-fetched that just knowing what's on a scan would affect your self-perception or your behavior. But I've had sixty-five-year-old patients who came to me with MRI scans already in hand, showing a bulging disc and asking what can be done about it. These people have no sign of a pinched nerve or serious disease on office examination. Remember that about 80 percent of people have a bulging disc at this age, even without pain. My efforts at reassurance have generally failed miserably.

Anecdotes aside, there's research showing that imaging results affect people's behavior. A British study enrolled people with back pain who had no sign of underlying infection, cancer, or nerve injury on an office examination. They were randomly assigned to get a spine X-ray or not. The people who got an X-ray were more satisfied with their care—but after several months they reported *more* pain and rated their health *worse* than the people who never got an X-ray. And they made more doctor visits.

Another study, done at the Cleveland Clinic, did MRI scans on a group of patients with back pain similar to those in the British study. But the researchers gave the results to only half the patients. When they were followed up later, once again the patients who got their results rated themselves less improved than the patients who never knew their results.

And what about the doctors who receive the imaging reports from the radiologist? Those bulging or degenerated discs can look like trouble to doctors, too. Scott Boden, the doctor from Emory University, warns, "A diagnosis that is based on magnetic resonance imaging, in the absence of objective clinical findings, may not be the cause of the patient's pain, and an attempt at operative correction could be the first step toward disaster."

That's doctor-speak for "Don't operate on the back just because you see something on the MRI." His caution is that there need to be abnormal findings on an office examination as well. Things like muscle weakness or missing reflexes, or pain on straight leg raising. Pain in the leg as well as pain in the back. Otherwise, fixing what's in the MRI picture may not help the patient and may just pose unnecessary risk.

Several years ago, we did a study that showed that this was more than a theoretical concern. Led once again by Dr. Jarvik, my neuroradiology colleague, we found patients whose doctors were sending them for plain X-rays of the spine. With the patients' and the doctors' consent, we randomly assigned them to get the X-ray as planned or to get an MRI instead. The MRI would show much more detailed information, but with the possibility of uncovering more irrelevant findings.

Sure enough, patients who got an MRI scan were twice as likely to have back surgery over the ensuing year. And despite twice as much surgery, the MRI group had exactly the same degree of improvement as the patients who got only a plain X-ray. There was a catch, though. Even though the medical results for the two groups were the same, those who got an MRI felt more satisfied with their care.

The finding that more imaging might result in more surgery is borne out by studies of geographic variations in care. If we look at small geographic regions, like cities, we see wide variations in rates of back surgery and also in rates of spine imaging. And where the rates of spine imaging are the highest, rates of back surgery are the highest.

These problems haven't restrained a rising tide of spine imaging tests in the U.S. When we examined Medicare claims, we found an increase of 307 percent in the number of low-back MRI scans done over twelve years, from 1994 to 2005. And yet over those years, patient surveys reported progressively worse problems with activity and function.

When you have back pain, you're going to be curious about what's causing it. The temptation to have a scan is almost irresistible. Friends and family may encourage it. But unless your doctor says there's a real need, don't push it. In this circumstance, knowledge isn't necessarily power; it's more often dangerous.

In fact, given research results like those I've described, the American College of Physicians and a group of family doctors have put spine imaging at the top of their lists of overused procedures. For low-risk patients, spine imaging is nearly always expense and risk without benefit. Instead, these professional groups urge doctors to order spine imaging only for high-risk patients who have "red flags" for unusual problems.

What are those red flags? What are the "extenuating circumstances" I mentioned at the start of this chapter? There are some very good reasons to get spine imaging, but they have little to do with severity of pain. They're things like having back pain along with a history of cancer, a history of injection drug abuse, unexplained fever, unexplained weight loss, or weakness in the leg or foot. They're things that a primary care doctor can identify in an office visit and might signal a serious underlying disease.

So spine imaging creates a conundrum. What we like—more tests—may not be what's best for us. Getting an imaging result is satisfying but may cause anxiety that makes things worse. And it's hard to celebrate the surgery you didn't have because you avoided an unnecessary MRI. Choosing wisely in this case is counterintuitive, but it may be the key to avoiding a cascade of unnecessary additional tests, treatments, and possible side effects.

In most cases, your doctor may recommend a course of treatment before considering any tests. The goal is to offer some pain relief while natural healing occurs, and this is usually feasible without any testing. What should that treatment consist of? Let's look at the example of prescription painkillers.

Chapter 4

PAINKILLERS

Easy Solutions Sometimes Aren't

earlier described David Fridovich as a tough guy. I called him that after reading his military history, reviewing his medical history, and talking to him. I'll tell you what I learned, and you can see if you agree with my description.

Recall that Fridovich was a college football star, Green Beret, and deputy commander of the nation's Special Forces. That includes the Green Berets, Army Rangers, Delta Force, Navy SEALS, and Air Force Rescue Teams. That's *Lieutenant General* Fridovich to you, but "Frido" to his close associates. Ten months before retiring in November 2011, Fridovich dropped a bombshell to reporters. He had struggled for five years with dependence on narcotic painkillers for chronic back pain.

After high school in Florida, Fridovich chose to attend Knox, a small college in Illinois. Fridovich says he chose Knox "to be independent and get out on my own. . . . I always had a dream to play some level of college football, and Knox would help me fulfill that dream." A three-year starting linebacker, Fridovich was voted co-captain and most valuable senior on the team. A former coach describes him as "the finest undergraduate leader" he can remember. Fridovich went on to complete a master's degree in political science at Tulane. He's now on the Board of Trustees at Knox.

Fridovich married his college sweetheart, Kathy, as he was about to enter the Army. He became a Green Beret and subsequently served as commander at every level in the Army: platoon, company, battalion, Special Forces Group, Special Operations Task Force, and Theater Special Operations Command. Along the way, he became assistant professor of military science at Norwich University, where he trained the Mountain Cold Weather Rescue Team.

Fridovich not only served at every level; he served all over the world. In 1995, he led a Special Operations Task Force in Haiti. His group helped to achieve a nearly bloodless transfer of power from the Haitian Army to elected officials. He later commanded a joint Special Operations Task Force in Sarajevo. In 2002, Fridovich led the training of counterterrorist forces in the Philippines. Later one of his Green Berets was the first American soldier killed in the Afghanistan war.

When Fridovich retired in 2011, commanders of the U.S. Special Operations were generous with their praise. Admiral Eric Olson said, "He is a man of action, whose operational excellence in many of the most remote, complex places on Earth earned him the ungrudging respect of his teams, his bosses, and his international colleagues . . . he gained the trust and cooperation and even the affection of the people of every place he went." Admiral Bill McRaven said of Fridovich, "His legacy as a Green Beret is unmatched—he is a leader in the army culture that values great warriors and equally great thinkers."

How did this accomplished man fall into the trap of narcotic dependence? Here we have details of a medical history because of Fridovich's self-disclosure.

After successful treatment, Fridovich disclosed his problem to the Army Vice Chief of Staff, General Peter Chiarelli, a four-star general. Fridovich says Chiarelli's jaw dropped. But shortly thereafter, Chiarelli called to ask if Fridovich would go public with his story. After a gasp, Fridovich said he would if it would help other soldiers.

I compiled the following description from the story Gregg Zoroya reported in *USA Today* in January 2011, an account by Adriana Colindres in the *Knox College Magazine*, and my own conversation with General Fridovich in 2012.

I'm going to avoid the term *narcotic* painkiller from here on, despite the virtue of its familiarity. For many, *narcotic* implies a disreputable or illegal substance. Though potentially dangerous, painkillers of the sort Fridovich used aren't illegal or disreputable. Instead, I'll use the more technical term, *opioid.*

Opioid describes a class of drugs similar to opium, hence the name. These medicines provide pain relief but also can cause dependency. Physical "dependency," which General Fridovich experienced, means that an unpleasant withdrawal syndrome occurs when a person stops using the drug. Used the wrong way, these medicines can also give a euphoric "high" and can lead to addiction—a form of more compulsive drug use. Someone can be *dependent* without showing signs of addiction. Some of these drugs are literally derived from opium and called opiates, but others are synthetic, hence the more generic term *opioids.*

The General's Back Pain

At about five feet nine inches tall, David Fridovich is not imposing in height, but he is solidly built. He has close-cropped thinning brown hair and big ears but is also broad shouldered. He's a devotee of physical conditioning and fitness.

Rather than a direct result of combat injury, General Fridovich's back pain began between trips to war zones. In 2006, he was working out doing leg presses at a Marine gym in Hawaii when he noticed a twinge in his back. In stoic form, he continued with weight training, racquetball, and handball for several days. Then one morning he awoke with pain from his lower back down his left leg. "All I could do was just lie in bed and writhe. . . . It felt like someone had taken a baseball bat from here to here," he told *USA Today*, pointing from his waist to his knee.

He reported to the emergency room at Tripler Army Medical Center in Honolulu. In our conversation, General Fridovich indicated that a key finding was a "grade I–II slip," referring to a substantial forward slip of one vertebra over the one below. This is called spondylolisthesis, but don't bother even trying to pronounce it. This problem can narrow the spinal canal and result in a pinched nerve, just as a herniated disc sometimes pinches a nerve. For General Fridovich, this sort of narrowing occurred along with degenerative changes in the discs that left "bone on bone."

Doctors initially treated him with Motrin and morphine. He then continued by taking Roxicet, a short-acting opioid, and OxyContin, a long-acting opioid. Fridovich described taking more than the prescribed doses because he was eager to resume his normal command activities. He reasoned that if the drugs were for pain relief, more drugs meant better relief.

In retrospect, Fridovich says, "What you find out is, the more you use, the less they work. You get saturated."

Furthermore, Fridovich encountered disturbing new symptoms. He described a foggy mind and frightening thoughts. He recalled, "That scared the hell out of me. Anxiety, depression, real bad thoughts."

So he cut back on the pills but didn't stop entirely. He continued with two to four pain pills a day, still commanding troops and advancing his career. As Fridovich told USA Today, "Somebody should have challenged me. I should have challenged myself and said, 'Wow, I'm on this stuff way too long. What's the deal?'"

By 2007, his wife, Kathy, was concerned about the medication. She said, "I knew he was taking a lot. I read all the little fine print. Drugs are scary." She urged her husband to find ways to stop. For a while, he underwent acupuncture to treat the pain—which "helped immensely"—and was able to reduce his use of opioids. But the pressures of regular travel to Afghanistan, Pakistan, and other hot spots meant that medication was the easiest way to manage the pain.

At this point, Fridovich thought the drugs—possibly along with the pain itself and the stresses of wartime—were responsible for personality changes. He queried colleagues in the Special Forces, where there's a reputation for blunt honesty, about his performance. They thought he was doing a great job. But Fridovich found himself being "in some ways, very isolated, very combative."

Later, when he finally reduced his opioid intake, Fridovich said his head cleared, his temperament eased, and his outlook improved. He joked to *USA Today*, "I should probably take an ad out in a national newspaper apologizing for everything I've said or done, because I'm a different person."

But before he reached that point, Fridovich would undergo yet further treatment for his back pain. In 2008, at Walter Reed Army Medical Center in Washington, D.C., a neurosurgeon performed a spinal fusion operation. Fridovich believes the surgery was critical for protecting his nerves from further injury, but his pain actually worsened afterward, so doctors escalated his opioid doses.

Finally, back home in Florida, a doctor had the temerity to tell the three-star general that he had a drug problem and needed a way to manage pain without the drugs. With help from a military health care program, Fridovich entered a special program in Pensacola, undergoing a month of physical training, psychological counseling, and detoxification.

"Detoxification" is partly a euphemism for withdrawal, which Fridovich described vividly. It left him "physically and emotionally wrung out after shakes, sweats, aches, and nausea." His summary was, "It's the most sickening feeling that racks your entire body." Strong words coming from the top Green Beret.

But the program introduced him to some new approaches to physical training and included a switch to a medication that's less subject to misuse, called buprenorphine. Massage helped with muscle tension. Therapists advised Fridovich to get more sleep and to abandon the macho military habit of five and a half hours a night.

Not only did his mood and thinking improve off the pain medication, but his pain actually improved. According to *USA Today*, at the end of the program, he recalls walking down stairs at home, smiling, and saying to his wife, "So this is what it feels like to be pain free."

In the end, Fridovich felt that the opioid medications had altered his personality, darkened his mood, worsened his management style, and strained his marriage. For such a high-ranking military officer to come forward with this type of personal problem was courageous. Fridovich could easily have kept these events part of his private life.

As a military colleague said, "Nobody wants to show weaknesses. You want to be perceived as perfection. . . . But sometimes moral courage kicks in where moral courage is demanded." General Chiarelli, who first encouraged Fridovich to go public, later said, "That guy is the bravest man I've ever met. . . . I don't think I've ever seen an act of leadership any greater than him doing what he did."

Fridovich came forward in part to dramatize a growing problem in the military. At the same time he revealed his story, he spoke to seven hundred military doctors and medics about an epidemic of chronic pain in the military and the risks of opioid pain relievers. *USA Today* noted that hospitalizations and diagnoses of substance abuse in the military had doubled in recent years.

An Army report estimated that up to a third of the ten thousand soldiers in wounded-care companies were dependent on or addicted to opioids. Only 10 percent of soldiers in these units have combat wounds; the remainder have other injuries, illnesses, or mental health concerns. Case managers and nurses estimated that 25 to 35 percent of soldiers in these units were "over-medicated, abuse prescriptions and have access to illegal drugs."

General Fridovich continues to share his story about opioid dependency, speaking at meetings on military and veteran health care.

Lessons from a General's Back Problems

What can we learn from the story of General Fridovich's struggle with dependency on painkillers? First, this isn't a problem that's confined to homeless drug addicts, whiners, goldbrickers, or teenagers seeking cheap thrills. Fridovich is a genuine tough guy with an unstoppable work ethic. He was a standout in a tough crowd.

A quick glance at the daily news tells us that Fridovich's predicament isn't so unusual. A host of prominent personalities have struggled with opioid dependence and even addiction, a situation that goes well beyond Fridovich's experience.

Cindy McCain, the wife of Senator John McCain, became addicted to Vicodin and Percocet, both opioid painkillers, after undergoing back surgery. The problem progressed to the point that she obtained illegal prescriptions before her parents recognized the problem and intervened. Dealing with patients who are dependent on opioids has evolved into a daily, challenging, and often frustrating problem for nearly every primary care doctor. Of course, the frustrations for patients are even worse.

Second, Fridovich did what so many patients do. He assumed that if some opioids are good, more must be better. He acknowledged increasing the doses beyond what his doctors prescribed. Many people assume that prescribed drugs, unlike street drugs, must be perfectly safe. So taking them, and increasing the dose, must be harmless. As we'll see, this is a dangerous assumption.

Also like many patients, Fridovich found it hard—really hard—to stop using opioids. Outright addiction is only a small part of the problem. The reality is that many people find it difficult to stop taking opioids, and researchers are still exploring the reasons. Some patients like the way they feel while taking opioid medications, and that makes stopping a challenge. But seeking a "high" doesn't seem to be the most frequent problem. More commonly, people develop tolerance to the pain-relieving effects of opioids over time and require increasing doses to get the same pain relief. This can lead to prolonged use and an increasing risk of side effects.

Other people develop a paradoxical *increase* in pain sensitivity while taking prescription opioids. This seems to be a result of changes in the nerve cells and the connections between them in the brain and spinal cord. It's as if the body overcompensates for having painkillers on board by turning up its sensitivity to painful events. This may lead to requests for yet more pain medication.

Furthermore, many people who use opioids for more than a few weeks become physically dependent. They may not get high, but they suffer withdrawal symptoms if they decrease the medication. That's what Fridovich described as feeling "physically and emotionally wrung out, after shakes, sweats, aches, and nausea." We might add restlessness, irritability, insomnia, and diarrhea to the list of common withdrawal symptoms. Nobody wants those symptoms, and continuing opioids is the path of least resistance.

In Fridovich's case, doctors started opioids from the beginning of the pain. Fridovich says the medications were helpful at the outset, and he was grateful for some relief. In retrospect, though, he wishes he had stopped opioids after a few weeks and started other pain control strategies.

Most guidelines today suggest that opioids aren't the first line of treatment for back pain, and a trial of non-opioid medications is often appropriate first. If opioids are used initially, a brief course is often best. If pain persists, non-drug treatments come to the fore, including physical therapy, exercise, relaxation techniques, and the like. As we'll see—and as the general's experience dramatizes—prolonged use of opioids for non-cancer pain may often be a bad idea.

Surgeons sometimes argue that back surgery is preferable to long-term opioid use and the resulting side effects. But it's rarely an "either-or" proposition. Fridovich continued using opioids beyond the immediate post-surgery healing period. The same thing happened to Cindy McCain. We might wonder if that was because of poor pain relief, drug dependence, or some combination. And it may be unclear even to patients and their doctors.

In any case, surgery didn't halt the use of painkillers. That may seem odd, but research suggests it's the norm. For example, among patients who had a spinal fusion operation in one prominent research study, more than eight out of ten were still taking opioids two years later.

Fridovich described dramatic mood changes that he attributed at least in part to opioid medications: frightening thoughts, anxiety, depression, and combativeness. In an individual case, it may be hard to be sure that these symptoms resulted from medication. The pain itself might be contributing, as well as the stresses of daily demands—of wartime duty, in Fridovich's case.

But the general thought they were at least partly drug-related, and other patients report similar symptoms. The mood changes affected other aspects of Fridovich's life. They worsened his management style and strained his marriage. Beyond mood, he described effects of opioids on his thinking—a foggy mind. This is another common complaint among patients receiving opioid therapy.

In the end, Fridovich felt better when doctors finally tapered his opioid medication. This may seem counterintuitive, but many patients report the same thing. Patients and doctors alike may assume that stopping opioids will worsen pain and diminish quality of life. Yet just the opposite often happens, once the patient is past the challenge of detoxification.

General Fridovich still has back pain every day and still takes buprenorphine. But his quality of life is good, and he doesn't believe that the pain—or any medication—is controlling his life. He has good days and bad days, but the pain is at a level he can cope with. He feels that he's had good medical care throughout his back problem and is grateful for the holistic approach that he's found so helpful.

At the end of our interview, he headed off to his regular exercise training session: sixty to ninety minutes a day of stretching, strength training, bicycling, and water resistance.

His advice to people with chronic back pain is, "Take ownership of the problem." He feels that it took time and a multidisciplinary approach to get himself on the right track. Denying the problem, assuming it will fix itself, or losing hope altogether are seductive approaches that he ultimately rejected.

Given these problems, it might be surprising that the prescribing of opioids for back pain has increased dramatically over the past fifteen years. Why has opioid prescribing become so popular?

Chapter 5

PAINKILLERS AND
THE MARKETING OF PAIN

Mood changes, foggy thinking, dependency, withdrawal. Feeling better once he stopped. The story of General David Fridovich illustrates the many drawbacks of long-term opioids for persistent back pain. Yet opioid prescribing in the United States has soared since 1996. Sales of prescription opioids quadrupled between 1999 and 2010. We've become a country awash in opioids, and much of the flood is related to back pain.

In part, increased opioid prescribing resulted from concerns that doctors were undertreating people with cancer, terminal illness, or acute injuries. Experts in medical ethics and patient advocates were vocal about the need to improve pain control, and doctors responded.

But today those conditions account for just a small fraction of opioid prescribing. Instead, doctors most often prescribe opioids for problems like back pain and arthritis. And the largest quantity of opioids go to people with long-term pain rather than acute injuries.

For a small number of arthritis patients, low-dose opioids may be helpful for long-term therapy. But more than half the patients who regularly use prescription opioids have back pain. Here the benefits are far less clear, the doses often higher, and the side effects more bothersome.

Randomized trials are the strongest type of research on the efficacy of medical treatments. But there are only a few such trials of long-term opioids for back pain. Even these studies tracked patients for only four months or less. Yet patients often take opioids for years or decades.

What can we learn from these rather short back pain studies? That any advantage of opioids over other pain medicines is modest at best. And we're left with no strong information about the safety or effectiveness of opioids for long-term treatment of back pain.

In the longer run, opioid tolerance—waning effects that may result in a dose increase—may blunt any benefit for pain relief. Tolerance, along with dependence and increased pain sensitivity, make any benefit for long-term pain more dubious than for short-term pain. Surveys show that patients who take long-term opioids actually report worse pain—while taking opioids—than pain patients who don't.

Long-Term Opioid Side Effects

What about side effects? Until recently, the conventional wisdom was that there was no ceiling to the safe dose of opioids, as long as doctors increased the dose gradually. But new studies are showing that large doses of opioids increase the risk of overdose and death.

One reason is that opioids slow breathing to the point that it can stop altogether. This risk increases when someone adds alcohol or certain other drugs to the mix. Opioid-related deaths have quadrupled since 1999, in perfect parallel with prescription opioid sales. That meant 16,651 deaths in 2010 alone, far more than deaths from heroin and cocaine combined.

A story reported in the news illustrates both the short-term benefits and the deadly risks. At age twenty-eight, Steve Rummler had back and leg pain attributed to an irritated nerve. He put up with it for nine years. At age thirty-seven, he finally got a prescription for hydrocodone, an opioid used in medicines like Vicodin. He also got a prescription for clonazepam, a sedative drug similar to Valium.

Rummler got some pain relief, but it was short-lived. In a diary, he wrote about the drugs. "At first they were a lifeline. Now they are a noose around my neck." Four years after starting the medications, Rummler had lapsed into addiction. His family urged him into addiction treatment, and he completed two programs.

Just forty-five days after completing rehab, at age forty-three, Rummler was found dead. He still had prescriptions for hydrocodone and clonazepam, and police found empty pill bottles. The official cause of death was mixed drug toxicity caused by opioids and sedatives. This turns out to be a particularly dangerous combination.

Along with mortality, admissions to substance abuse treatment have increased 400 percent over the past decade. The most common reason—aside from marijuana—wasn't street drugs. It was prescription opioids. Emergency room visits for opioid abuse doubled in just four years. The White House Office of Drug Control Policy describes the current situation as an *epidemic* of prescription drug abuse.

Discussing death and overdose may seem like scare tactics. But consider some of the other, more common risks of long-term opioids. General Fridovich demonstrated some of opioid therapy's effects on mood and thinking. Studies of older adults show decreased short-term memory and response times. These in turn account for the higher likelihood of traffic accidents among seniors taking opioids. In pregnant women, opioids for pain can cause a withdrawal syndrome for the newborn baby.

Many people don't realize that long-term opioid use can lead to sexual problems. These include difficulty getting an erection and decreased sex drive for men. Testosterone levels fall rapidly after opioids are started. Those levels recover when the medicine stops but may stay low if it continues. In extreme cases, hormone changes in women can lead to infertility. Patient information brochures often refer to these problems with vague terms like "endocrine dysfunction" without spelling out what that means.

In older adults, opioid therapy increases falls, fractures, and osteoporosis. Persistent constipation is common and can even lead to bowel obstruction. Researchers have attributed a litany of other problems to opioid therapy, and the full range of complications is still under study.

How Did We Get into an Epidemic of Prescription Opioid Abuse?

Dr. Jane Ballantyne is an internationally renowned specialist in pain medicine. Originally from England, she trained in surgery and in anesthesiology in Oxford. She then moved to the United States and did more training in pain medicine at Boston's prestigious Massachusetts General Hospital. This is one of Harvard's primary teaching hospitals. She has major editorial roles in prominent medical journals concerning pain research and in one of the definitive textbooks of pain management. In 2012, she was one of the country's "top doctors" in *U.S. News* ratings.

Dr. Ballantyne is an outspoken critic of the way doctors currently prescribe opioids. She recently wrote, "We are providing a treatment that for many patients is not improving their pain but is compromising their lives and futures."

If there's little long-term benefit of opioids for treating back pain, and clear evidence of harm, why has prescribing quadrupled in recent years? Listen to Dr. Ballantyne: "Who taught us to do all this? In large part, it has been the drug companies that have for years picked the message and the messengers while sponsoring much of the postgraduate education and all the major pain meetings."

What's in it for the drug industry? In 2011, the market for prescription opioids was $8.4 billion, according to a company that tracks medication use. And the single most prescribed drug in the United States is hydrocodone—the drug Steve Rummler took.

How do drug companies influence doctors' conferences and educational programs? One of the medical societies that provides such programs, the American Academy of Pain Medicine (AAPM), lists members of its "Corporate Relations Council" on its website. The society notes,

"They receive premiere status at AAPM's Annual Meeting and other networking events."

"Premiere status" includes the opportunity to produce sponsored seminars attached to the meetings. The member list includes such companies as Purdue Pharma, Abbott Laboratories, and Endo Pharmaceuticals, the makers of OxyContin, Vicodin, and Percodan, respectively. The same companies appear as Corporate Council Members of the American Pain Society.

It's perfectly legal for drug companies to support doctors' groups, of course. But as Dr. Ballantyne suggests, recent events raise concern about the companies' influence on medical organizations and doctors' prescribing habits.

This came to a head in 2012, when the Senate Finance Committee announced an investigation into ties among the makers of opioid painkillers, doctors' groups, and some patient advocacy groups.

Those ties are strong. According to news reports, for example, the American Academy of Pain Medicine received $1.3 million from the drug industry in 2011. The American Pain Society received $1.6 million over two years. In 2010, the American Pain Foundation, a patient advocacy group, received about $4.5 million from drug and medical device companies. That constituted 90 percent of the organization's budget. The American Pain Foundation closed its doors the night the Finance Committee announced its investigation.

Senators Max Baucus (D-Montana) and Charles Grassley (R-Iowa) from the Finance Committee seemed to share Dr. Ballantyne's concerns. They sent letters requesting financial records and communications to several drug makers and doctors' organizations, including Purdue Pharma, Endo Pharmaceuticals, the American Academy of Pain Medicine, and the American Pain Society. Their letters referred to the epidemic of opioid abuse: "There is growing evidence pharmaceutical companies that manufacture and market opioids may be responsible, at least in part, for this epidemic by promoting misleading information about the drugs' safety and effectiveness."

Some experts date the greatest increase in opioid prescribing to 1996, when the FDA approved OxyContin. This was a new, long-acting preparation of an older drug called oxycodone. Purdue Pharma introduced the new medicine with an inspired marketing campaign. The marketing was not just advertising but included more stealthy promotion strategies as well.

For example, a 2003 report from the General Accounting Office (GAO) pointed to Purdue Pharma's partnership with the Joint Commission on Accreditation of Healthcare Organizations, often just called the "Joint Commission." The report described the partnership as a strategy that "facilitated access to hospitals to promote OxyContin." The Joint Commission sets standards for care and reviews U.S. hospitals on a recurring basis. Hospital administrators fear these accreditation visits and take them very seriously. You couldn't ask for a better way to get people's attention.

In addition, the American Pain Society and the Joint Commission promoted the concept of "pain as the fifth vital sign," a phrase trademarked by the pain society. The idea was to ask patients to rate their pain at every doctor visit, like checking the pulse or blood pressure.

The intent may have been well meaning. But many doctors saw the tracking of pain scores at every visit as a spur to prescribe opioids. This was the fastest and easiest way to deal with pain complaints. And by prescribing, doctors would prove to both patients and administrators that they were taking pain complaints seriously. Doctors today often have part of their incomes tied to patient satisfaction surveys, and some doctors feel pressured to prescribe opioids to maintain high patient satisfaction.

The GAO report also noted that Purdue Pharma "funded over 20,000 pain-related educational programs through direct sponsorship or financial grants." These programs included the hospital "grand rounds" presentations attended by many doctors, as well as educational seminars at state and local medical conferences.

In 1996, the year of OxyContin's debut, the American Pain Society and the American Academy of Pain Medicine formed a guideline panel that supported long-term opioid therapy. The statement indicated that the risk of addiction was low, that breathing complications were rare, that waning effectiveness was uncommon, and that fears of drug diversion shouldn't limit prescribing. Purdue Pharma helped support the guideline panel, which was headed by Dr. David Haddox. Purdue Pharma later hired Dr. Haddox.

Purdue Pharma's marketing and education about OxyContin were sometimes less than factual. A decade later, Purdue Pharma's top three executives pled guilty to criminal charges that they "misled regulators, doctors and patients about the drug's risk of addiction and its potential to be abused." The company agreed to a $600 million settlement of civil and criminal charges. Courts sentenced the three executives to probation in lieu of jail time and barred them from doing business with Medicare or Medicaid.

Purdue Pharma wasn't the only company accused of misleading marketing. In 2008, Cephalon reached a settlement for alleged illegal marketing of three drugs, including Actiq. Actiq is a strong opioid painkiller produced in the form of a lollipop. The FDA approved it only for use by cancer patients who no longer responded to other opioids. But the company allegedly promoted it for patients with non-cancer pain and without the loss of responsiveness. Cephalon ultimately paid a $425 million settlement.

The combined overt and stealthy marketing activities had an impact. Doctors came to see long-term opioid prescribing for chronic non-cancer pain as routine treatment. They were much quicker to prescribe opioids than they had been in the past. The prescribing was well intentioned and was driven by a desire to provide compassionate care. Indeed, a strong message was that it would be unethical to do otherwise. Professional societies, accrediting agencies, and respected experts in pain management broadcast the message widely.

But no one conveyed the message that there was virtually no evidence to support the efficacy or safety of the drugs for long-term use. It was the back business at its busiest.

How much effect does prescription painkiller abuse have on our society? One research group used data from insurance claims, federal surveys, criminal justice reports, and the Bureau of Labor Statistics to come up with an estimate. They concluded that abuse or dependence on prescription painkillers cost society about $56 billion in 2007. Of that total, about $5 billion was for criminal justice costs, and the remainder was evenly split between health care costs and workplace costs.

In retrospect, one vocal doctor argued, "Untreated chronic pain is a serious problem. But opioids are rarely the answer. Chronic pain patients need and deserve compassionate care and evidence-based treatment."

Others have recently summarized that there's little evidence that opioids are more effective than other treatments for persistent pain; that dependence and addiction are far more common than doctors and patients realize; and that doctors often prescribe a larger supply than necessary. They concluded, "It is time to collectively lower expectations and prescribe these drugs less readily, to fewer patients, at lower doses, and for shorter periods."

Of course, opioid painkillers have been around a long time. Opium has been used since antiquity. What about newer drugs for treating pain?

Chapter 6

PAIN MANAGEMENT,
NOW THAT'S MONEY

You may imagine that the marketing of opioid painkillers was uniquely aggressive. But company marketing of other drugs for pain has followed a similar path. Some other marketing stories may make you wonder if drug makers are exploiting people desperate for relief.

The story of Vioxx is now a familiar example. Vioxx was a nonsteroidal anti-inflammatory drug, or NSAID, that was widely sold for painful conditions like back pain. Ibuprofen, naproxen, and others belong to the same class of drugs. Recall that the manufacturer, Merck, withdrew Vioxx from the market in 2004 because it increased the risk of heart attacks and strokes.

An FDA scientist estimated that Vioxx caused about one hundred forty thousand avoidable heart attacks. Several studies combined showed that the risk of a heart attack with Vioxx was about twice the risk with similar drugs or with placebo.

Other researchers found that most who took Vioxx would have done just as well with much cheaper ibuprofen. That's the drug in common remedies such as Advil and Motrin. Ibuprofen appeared to be just as effective as Vioxx, whose main advantage was less stomach irritation. But most patients who took Vioxx had no risk factors for serious stomach irritation or bleeding. Yet Vioxx was earning $2.5 billion a year before Merck pulled it from the market.

Thousands of people who used Vioxx sued the manufacturer, claiming the drug had caused heart attacks or strokes. In 2007, Merck settled 26,000 cases for almost $5 billion. A year later, the company settled claims of deceptive advertising for $58 million. A few years later, it settled criminal and civil charges for another $1 billion. The federal prosecutor cited unsupported safety claims among the charges.

Merck used several strategies to promote the drug aside from ubiquitous TV and print ads aimed at the public. It pushed doctors to prescribe the drug. To this end, the company paid for scientific articles to be ghostwritten and attributed to prominent medical school faculty members. It undertook so-called seeding trials, which looked like legitimate research but were intended to get more doctors to prescribe Vioxx. In essence, "research" of this sort creates an opportunity to pay doctors to prescribe a drug and to get more comfortable prescribing it.

And there were accusations that the company tried to hush doctors who spoke out about the risks of Vioxx. The story of Dr. Gurkipal Singh, as told by Snigdha Prakash on National Public Radio, is instructive. Prakash used internal company emails and other communications that became available as court documents.

As Vioxx became available, Merck sought influential doctors to speak at medical seminars. Among others, the company recruited Dr. Gurkipal Singh, an arthritis specialist at Stanford University. Dr. Singh gave some forty lectures related to Vioxx over seven months.

But as concerns about heart attack risks began to emerge, Dr. Singh asked the company to show him the findings. According to NPR, the company promised to provide study results to Dr. Singh but never delivered. Dr. Singh began to mention concern about this side effect in his lectures, which were monitored by local sales representatives and doctors friendly to the company.

As Singh began to discuss the possible heart side effects, the company wanted to stop him from lecturing. A sample internal document read, "At nine meetings in LA area over the past three days, Singh presented sessions that were very unfavorable to Vioxx." An e-mail from a Merck marketing manager said, "Dr. Singh continues to play up the CV [cardiovascular] events associated with Vioxx . . . we have many other speakers who deliver good messages, and we should not risk supporting the negative messages that he continues to deliver."

Merck executives conferred on how to rein in Dr. Singh. E-mails suggested that they wanted to quiet his voice but were afraid of alienating him. At the same time, some participants in the discussions acknowledged that the concerns were legitimate. Finally, a dossier was prepared for a Merck senior vice-president who was an influential doctor.

Singh's immediate boss at Stanford was Dr. Jim Fries. Fries recalled getting a call on a Saturday from the Merck vice-president, indicating, "Someone on my staff was making wild and irresponsible public statements about cardiovascular side effects of Vioxx." A later e-mail by the vice-president said, "Fries and I discussed getting Singh to stop making outrageous comments. . . . I will keep the pressure on and get others at Stanford to help."

The vice-president advised a marketing director, "Tell Singh we've told his boss about his Merck-bashing. And tell him, 'should it continue, further actions will be necessary (don't define it).'" Similar calls were made to other medical schools. When confronted with this evidence, Merck argued that it was just maintaining balance in a vigorous public debate.

Another interpretation might be that the company was desperately trying to suppress bad news. In the end, though, research on the risks of Vioxx finally overwhelmed the company's efforts.

Vioxx was a drug that had little advantage over older drugs, and worse side effects.

Other new drugs have been promoted for treating conditions like back pain when there simply was little evidence that they worked.

This was the situation for Neurontin, a drug the FDA first approved in 1993 as adjunctive therapy for an unusual form of seizures. That means it was only to be used as a secondary drug along with other seizure medications. Later the FDA also approved Neurontin for treating pain after an episode of herpes zoster, also known as shingles.

If these sound to you like fairly unusual medical situations, and a pretty small market, you'd be right. So how did Neurontin come to have almost $3 billion a year in sales by 2004?

The manufacturer of Neurontin was Parke-Davis, a subsidiary of Warner-Lambert, now owned by Pfizer. Parke-Davis undertook a campaign to expand Neurontin's rather small market by promoting it for psychiatric conditions and for other types of pain. Neurontin is now often known by its generic name, gabapentin.

A young biologist, Dr. David Franklin, went to work for Parke-Davis in 1996 and became a whistle-blower in the marketing campaign. Franklin claimed the company illegally influenced and provided kickbacks to doctors for using Neurontin—for purposes never approved by the FDA.

As long as a drug has at least one FDA-approved use, such "off-label" prescribing is legal, based on a doctor's judgment. But it's illegal for companies to market drugs for these off-label uses.

A Parke-Davis executive reportedly told Franklin shortly after he was hired, "I want you out there every day selling Neurontin. . . . We all know Neurontin's not growing for adjunctive therapy, besides that's not where the money is. Pain management, now that's money."

The executive went on to describe ways to influence doctors, including "one-on-one . . . holding their hand and whispering in their ear, Neurontin for pain . . . Neurontin for everything. . . . I don't want to hear that safety crap, either."

How would a company representative whisper in a doctor's ear? The federal suit that followed the whistle-blower suit alleged that Parke-Davis paid doctors $350 a day to allow sales representatives to join them as they saw patients.

Court documents described a memo to Parke-Davis sales representatives instructing them to offer promising doctors an expenses-paid weekend at a Florida resort and a $250 honorarium. A voicemail message from one manager to sales reps said, "When we get [to doctors], we want to kick some ass. We want to sell Neurontin on pain. All right?"

The suit also claimed that the company paid key doctors $1,000 each to attach their names to ghostwritten scientific articles that recommended Neurontin for unapproved uses. Other doctors were paid as speakers for medical seminars, with one earning $300,000 over three years. The so-called off-label uses of Neurontin—like treating back pain—came to account for 90 percent of its sales.

Did the company have research showing that Neurontin was effective for back pain? Internal documents show that the company undertook six research studies for so-called nociceptive pain, a term it used to include back pain. However, the documents show that only one had a positive result, and the other five showed no benefit from Neurontin. Perhaps it's no surprise that none of these studies was ever published.

University researchers who reviewed the court documents found that the company undertook these studies for the clear purpose of encouraging off-label use of Neurontin. Company officials called this their "publication strategy," as opposed to an FDA approval strategy.

Given the marketing purpose of the company-sponsored studies, the company published its results whenever they suggested Neurontin worked but avoided publishing if the results showed no benefit. There were some positive results for conditions other than nociceptive pain.

But if the results showed no benefit, the company either didn't publish them at all or found a way to put a favorable spin on them. The university researchers were concerned that this approach did "not meet the ethical standards for clinical research or maintain the integrity of scientific knowledge."

In the end, the company—now owned by Pfizer—agreed to plead guilty of "false claims" and to pay $430 million for criminal and civil charges.

To this day, is there any scientific evidence that Neurontin, or its generic version, gabapentin, is effective for treating back pain? An extensive review turned up very few studies and concluded there was nothing to recommend this medication for back pain.

There are all too many other examples of "advances" for treating back pain that turned out not to be. But of the many choices, let's consider just one more: a product intended for injection rather than a pill. In fact, a product intended to provide mechanical support rather than systemwide effects. Here we take a digression from the common type of back pain, where the underlying diagnosis is often unclear, to a more specific cause of back pain.

For people with osteoporosis, usually older adults, an occasional complication is partial collapse of a vertebra. Doctors call this a compression fracture. These events aren't always painful, and sometimes people are unaware that they even happened. But sometimes they are painful, and people seek pain relief.

A new procedure in the past fifteen years involves injecting bone "cement" into the affected vertebrae. Doctors hope this will alleviate pain and prevent further collapse. They also hope to avoid the hunchback—or "dowager's hump"—that can result from multiple compression fractures.

In its simple form, the procedure is called a vertebroplasty. Here the doctor injects cement under pressure directly into the center of a vertebra. A more complex version involves inflating a "balloon" inside the vertebra before injection, to make a space in the bone marrow for the cement. The balloon may also perhaps slightly expand the collapsed vertebra. This is called a kyphoplasty procedure.

Most often, doctors inject the same cement they use to fix artificial hip or knee joints in place, called methyl methacrylate. But the growing market for vertebroplasty materials prompted new entries into the bone cement market. One of these was a material named Norian XR, made by the biotech company Norian, itself a subsidiary of a company called Synthes.

In slightly different forms, the Norian product was already approved by the FDA for use in the arm and in the skull. But company officials saw a larger market for use of Norian XR in vertebroplasty. The FDA posed a speed bump, though, indicating that use in the spine would almost certainly require new clinical research, involving plenty of time and many patients. One estimate was three years and $1 million for such a project.

We have details of company decisions from employee interviews, court transcripts, and documents submitted in a criminal case against Synthes. Mina Kimes summarized the events at length in *Fortune* magazine.

After the discouraging response from the FDA, Synthes made a fateful decision. Rather than launch a formal research study, the company began market research with spine surgeons.

Some surgeons began using Norian in vertebroplasty procedures, but two of the earliest patients had major complications. They had drastic falls in blood pressure shortly after the cement was injected. The doctors providing anesthesia had to give emergency drugs to avoid disaster.

Despite these early warnings, company officials made a decision "to get a few sites to perform 60–80 procedures and help them publish their clinical results." This could help to popularize use of the cement. The company also applied for FDA approval using an approach that would not require clinical studies. Companies often use this approach when modifying products that the FDA has already approved.

According to *Fortune*, the FDA granted approval for use of Norian XR in the spine, but with an important restriction. Doctors were not to mix it with anything else before injecting. Unfortunately, mixing the material with barium sulfate was exactly what vertebroplasty procedures required.

Furthermore, in animal studies, small amounts of Norian cement in the bloodstream caused rapid, severe blood clotting and death. In humans, this might occur if some of the cement leaked during a vertebroplasty.

Fortune reported that despite misgivings by some employees at Synthes, the plan to test Norian XR in humans proceeded, with the rationale that it was simply an off-label use. Things went well for a few dozen procedures, and the FDA approved general use of the mixed product in the spine, but again with an important restriction. Norian XR was *not* to be used for vertebroplasty. In fact, the FDA required a specific warning on the label saying that Norian was not intended for treating vertebral compression fractures.

Nonetheless, some surgeons were still interested in Norian XR for vertebroplasty. Sales reps continued to train surgeons in its use. All who were involved still used the rationale that it was an off-label use, but perhaps effective.

A month after FDA approval for use of the mixed product in the spine, a Texas surgeon undertook the procedure in a seventy-year-old woman, Lois Eskind. Just seconds after the surgeon injected the cement, Ms. Eskind had a dramatic fall in blood pressure. Attempts to resuscitate her continued unsuccessfully for thirty minutes, and she died.

Nonetheless, *Fortune* reports, Synthes staffers proceeded to develop a sales plan for Norian XR in the spine. They projected a $20 million market within two years, with a profit margin of 50 percent after taxes.

But a few months later, prize-winning physicist Ryoichi Kikuchi died on the operating table. Again, this occurred after a plunge in blood pressure. In spite of the deaths, a Synthes executive approved a technical brochure for surgeons that omitted the FDA warning against using Norian for vertebroplasty.

After yet another death in the operating room, the FDA began to investigate a tip about off-label marketing. Thus began five years of investigation and grand jury hearings that led to criminal charges against Norian, Synthes, and four top executives. At least five operating room deaths had occurred after Norian XR was injected for vertebroplasty.

In the end, the U.S. Attorney's office issued a press release alleging that Synthes had engaged in "human experimentation." In 2010, Synthes pleaded guilty, agreed to $23 million in fines, and agreed to divest Norian.

A judge sentenced each of the four Synthes executives to several months of prison time. This is one of the few examples of punishing corporate leaders with incarceration. The sentencing judge declared, "What has occurred in this case, in terms of wrongfulness—it's 11 on a scale of 10."

Nonetheless, some family members of the deceased patients argued that the sentences were "piddly." *Fortune* described the daughter of one patient who said, "They could have gone to 7-Eleven and stolen a six-pack of beer and got more time." The families of some of the patients are still pursuing civil suits.

Digging a little deeper, newer research has challenged the value of vertebroplasty with any kind of bone cement. That detail aside, the story of Norian is an extreme case of skirting the law to promote treatments that have dubious value or are even harmful. It's a reminder that newer isn't always better, and provides a cautionary tale for anyone seeking to jump the gun to get the latest and greatest.

If medications for back pain have sometimes proved disappointing, would surgery be a better choice?

Chapter 7

STABBED IN THE BACK

After a nagging pain began in his right hip, Dr. Jerome Groopman couldn't stop exercising—he was training for the Boston Marathon. His doctor prescribed "taking it easy" but acquiesced to Groopman's suggestion that he could at least work out on a rowing machine. After a few minutes on the rowing machine—set at high resistance—"a viselike spasm exploded" in Groopman's lower back. "Electric shocks raced down my legs. I fell to the floor. It took many hours, lying in a fetal position, until the pain eased."

Advised by both his physician wife and a sports orthopedist to take anti-inflammatory medicine, rest, and wait, Groopman was impatient. He told me he wishes that his wife had had a choke leash.

"I wanted an immediate remedy and stubbornly believed I knew what was best." After all, Groopman was himself a doctor, and one who'd recently finished about ten years of medical school, internship, residency, and a fellowship at three elite institutions. "Waiting patiently for nature to heal me seemed passive and paltry, so I doctor-shopped, seeking the second opinion I wanted to hear."

Two operations later, he was in unrelenting agony. Looking back after nineteen years, Groopman said, "I have never fully recovered from the surgery. Not a day passes when I don't fail to think of my head-strong decision, because of the limits on my function." Like John Kennedy, Dr. Groopman had a strong conviction that surgery was the best approach to his back pain but found that it was far from being a cure. Groopman described these events in the prologue to his book *Second Opinions*.

What went wrong?

Years later, Dr. Groopman is tall, thin, and balding but with a full, neatly trimmed white beard and owlish glasses. In short, the visage of a stereotypical college professor. And indeed, he is a medical school professor. He holds an endowed professorship at Harvard Medical School, where he's a specialist in cancer medicine, and he's chief of experimental medicine at the Beth Israel Deaconess Medical Center. He's a prolific medical researcher. He's a member of the Institute of Medicine, a prestigious organization with a highly select invited membership that often advises the government on medical issues.

But that's just half his career. The other half is as a literary writer. Aside from his prolific scientific articles, he's published five best-selling books related to medicine and biology. He's also a staff writer for the *New Yorker* and frequently pens editorials for the likes of the *New York Times* and the *Wall Street Journal*. My description of his back pain is possible because of his writings and an interview we conducted in 2013.

If ever there was a smart, well-informed consumer and patient, Groopman must have been it. How could he, of all people, fall into the trap of ineffective therapy—or worse?

After doctor-shopping in search of the second opinion he wanted to hear, Groopman found a neurosurgeon willing to do an operation for a "nerve pinched by a bulging lumbar disc." From that description, it sounds like a genuine herniated disc. Thirty years later, we may never know. But remember that imaging tests aren't perfect and don't show pain. It's at least possible—as with President Kennedy—that the disc wasn't really the culprit.

Removing a disc to relieve a pinched nerve is called a "decompression" operation because it relieves compression on the nerve.

Sometimes nerves get pinched by the bones themselves, as in the case of General Fridovich. Sometimes other structures in the spinal canal can pinch a nerve. Any operation to relieve the pressure on a nerve—by removing parts of a disc, a bone, or a ligament—can be called a decompression.

In any event, after surgery, Groopman still had aching in his back and hip. He felt better but still restricted. One day, standing up after coffee at a friend's house, he once again experienced severe pain in his low back and "electric shocks" down his legs.

Ordinarily, surgery for a herniated disc is pretty successful. It's aimed at removing the part of the disc that's pinching the nerve. But this type of surgery is better at relieving leg pain than back pain. It's common to hear doctors quote a 90 percent success rate, which sounds awfully good.

It's important to realize, though, that disc surgery isn't a panacea. Many patients, like Dr. Groopman, continue to have some discomfort even after surgery. Sometimes the same disc can herniate again, and sometimes another disc herniates. Sometimes scarring causes persistent pain. Sometimes leg pain goes away but back pain persists.

Sometimes the disc may be a red herring and not the actual cause of the pain. Today Dr. Groopman acknowledges the uncertainty we described earlier: the weak relationship between imaging results and what actually causes the pain. He calls this a "rupture of the cause and effect relationship" we've come to expect from modern medicine.

Furthermore, that success rate for surgery tells us nothing about the success rate of nonsurgical treatment, which is also very high. It's just that nonsurgical improvement is slower. Surgery gives faster relief, but after a year or two, or three, randomized trials suggest the results are similar.

Many patients and doctors assume that a herniated disc means you won't get better without surgery. But in fact, the usual course is favorable, even if recovery is slow. Remember in the chapter on spine imaging that we found herniated discs usually shrink on their own over a matter of months.

So this is one of those areas of medicine where there's a real choice. Some patients, given severe back pain and sciatica, would give anything for immediate relief, happily accept the risks of surgery, and waste no time going under the knife. Eager to run the Boston Marathon, Dr. Groopman made that choice.

But given what we know, other patients might conclude, "Well, if I can gradually improve without surgery, I'd prefer that. Surgery scares me, and if my doctor will help me with pain relief in the meantime, I'd rather wait and see if I get better on my own. I can put up with it." And surgery remains an option if that improvement never occurs.

Consider the experience of another doctor, Sam Ho. About a decade ago, Dr. Ho, chief medical officer of a California insurance company, developed sudden, severe back pain. Imaging tests showed a major herniated disc. Dr. Ho told the *New York Times* that he consulted a neurosurgeon, who insisted that he needed a laminectomy—a decompression operation to remove the disc. But his surgeon couldn't provide studies proving the operation would help, couldn't say how many operations he had done, or offer any data on his own patients' results. Dr. Ho declined the surgery and recovered nicely over the next two months.

So surgery and nonsurgical treatment are both choices a reasonable person might make when faced with a herniated disc. In this kind of case, your preferences really matter. This is an example where you, the patient, need to be well informed and involved in the decision making.

What happened to Dr. Groopman when the back pain and electric shocks came back? He reports that imaging tests didn't show any bulging discs this time around. He saw neurosurgeons, sports medicine doctors, and joint specialists, all of whom counseled patience.

But Groopman describes himself as "emotionally frayed and bitterly frustrated by the lack of answers. The cause of my problem had to be defined and aggressive solutions applied. I was determined to be permanently repaired." This is surely how many people would respond to a similar situation.

Once again, he kept searching for the opinion he wanted to hear. Finally, an orthopedic surgeon in Beverly Hills told Groopman that he had "instability" of the lower spine and needed a spine fusion operation. The surgeon cheerfully predicted that Groopman would be running within two weeks.

Having a Second Back Operation

Spinal fusion is quite different from a decompression operation, though they're often combined. In spine fusion surgery, the idea is to "weld" two or more vertebrae together with bone grafts. Eventually, as the bone grafts heal, the vertebrae essentially fuse into one longer bone. It's a bit like creating an internal brace.

Traditionally, surgeons take bone for grafting from the ridge of the pelvic bone, and that's what happened in Groopman's case. Today there are more options, but the principle is the same.

All back surgery, though, isn't the same. Fusion surgery is a bigger operation than removing a herniated disc. The surgeon has to dissect the muscles away from the bones he plans to fuse, remove some of the hard bony surface from the vertebrae, and place the bone fragments that will eventually heal to connect the vertebrae. If the surgeon removes bone from the pelvis, there may be another incision.

In most cases today, the surgeon will also insert screws with connecting rods or plates to hold the vertebrae in place while the bone heals. That's tricky work that requires the placement and angle of the screws to be just right. Compared with removing part of a disc, a fusion operation takes longer, causes more blood loss, and results in a higher complication rate. It's not like getting a haircut, and it's frightfully expensive.

Given the costs and risks of spine surgery, and especially fusion operations, you might imagine that doctors concur on when they need to perform a fusion. You might imagine that if they evaluated the same patients, surgeons would all agree on what type of surgery they should do. But you'd be wrong.

Doctors at Dartmouth Medical School have for decades studied variability in the way doctors use medical treatments. They've found that for many operations, if you compare rates of surgery among small geographic areas, there are surprising differences. Spine surgery shows some of the greatest variation among regions. For example, in 2010, for every one thousand people in Medicare, Wyoming did six times more in-hospital surgery than Hawaii. Oregon did two and a half times more surgery than New Jersey. Rates of spine fusion surgery vary even more than simpler forms of back surgery.

Does that mean people have weaker spines in Wyoming and Oregon? Seems unlikely. Most studies of back pain and herniated discs conclude that they occur at about the same rate wherever you look. Are people in Oregon and Wyoming just whiners? That seems unlikely, too.

Maybe it's because there are so many cowboys in Oregon and Wyoming, but not in Hawaii or New Jersey. But actually, cowboy isn't such a common occupation anymore. And surgery rates aren't closely linked to local occupations.

The Dartmouth researchers think that much of the variation in surgery rates is because doctors *don't agree* on who needs surgery or what kind. Surveys and other research back up that idea.

Dr. Bob Hart, my orthopedic colleague who studied President Kennedy's back problems, has also studied differences in decision making among spine surgeons. He did this by presenting several neurosurgeons and orthopedic surgeons with a series of detailed patient descriptions, complete with MRI scans, and asking what they would recommend. There were considerable differences of opinion among the surgeons. There were disagreements about who needed surgery, and disagreements about what kind of surgery was appropriate. Other studies have reported similar results.

Back in Boston, Dr. Jeff Katz studied which patients undergoing spine surgery had a fusion and which ones simply had a decompression without a fusion. Katz is a Harvard professor of rheumatology, the specialty that deals with joints and arthritis. He found that a decision to perform a fusion related more to surgeon preference than to any differences he could find among the patients.

More recently, a neurosurgeon reported her experience with providing second opinions for 183 patients who were told they needed spine surgery. In her opinion, 61 percent of the recommended operations were unnecessary, and another 33 percent were the wrong operation. The "wrong" procedures were typically more extensive than necessary.

So bear in mind that the decision to perform back surgery, and especially fusion surgery, is often not cut and dried. The chair of orthopedic surgery at my institution says, "If you're willing to get another opinion to remodel your bathroom, shouldn't you do the same for your spine?"

In fact, when Dr. Groopman decided to have a fusion operation, he was aware that his surgeon's practice partner was not so enthusiastic about the operation. But, he said, "I was not deterred. The heady promise of the orthopedist made moot any other consideration."

Groopman now refers to his decision for surgery as the "seduction of a quick fix. It may sound too good to be true, but you want it to be true."

How did the fusion operation work out for Groopman?

He awoke from the anesthesia to find that moving his legs or flexing his toes "triggered waves of such pain that my previous symptoms seemed minor." He returned home in a body brace, iced his back for three months, and took Percodan and other opioid painkillers. Groopman says these left him "nauseated and dopey" and made it hard to focus or think—and he still had relentless pain in his back, buttocks, and legs.

His orthopedic surgeon attributed the pain to scarring around the nerves and recommended another operation to free the nerves. This time, Groopman followed his wife's advice to decline.

Groopman eventually started physical therapy and stopped the opioids, but he reports that his therapy was largely passive; the therapists slowly moved his legs up and down. In a warm pool with parallel bars, he gradually began walking again. He says he was "disgusted with myself for undergoing the fusion surgery."

Groopman was able to return to work but continued having pain and kept a cot in his laboratory to lie on. He describes often lying on the floor to relieve pain during the conferences that follow hospital rounds with medical students and residents.

For nineteen years, he severely limited his activities. He couldn't swing a baseball bat with his sons and limited his evening walks with his wife. He went for a spine MRI that failed to render an explanation of his pain.

Groopman describes the next chapter of his story in his later best-selling book, *The Anatomy of Hope*. Eventually, a rheumatologist persuaded Groopman to see Dr. James Rainville, a rehabilitation doctor at the New England Baptist Hospital—the same hospital where John Kennedy had his first disc operation.

We'll pick up that story later, as we discuss exercise therapy. But let's pause here to consider Groopman's surgical adventures.

Lessons from a Doctor's Back Pain

Dr. Groopman's experience, like that of President Kennedy, reminds us that surgery is no panacea for back pain. Failure of other treatments is not an indication for back surgery. Surgery works best when there's a clear-cut anatomical abnormality that explains clear-cut findings on an office examination.

Although Groopman apparently had a herniated disc at the time of his initial surgery, it's possible that was a red herring, as we've learned is common. As we've also seen, most people with pain from a herniated disc can recover even without surgery. Like many of us, though, Groopman was in a hurry to get better, and he acknowledged his own impatience.

At the time of his second operation, the diagnosis was considerably less clear. Dr. Groopman now acknowledges this himself. He wrote, "In hindsight, I blamed myself more than the surgeons: I had pressed them for a solution when, in fact, none was apparent because the cause of the pain was obscure."

Several specialists advised against another operation, perhaps based on lack of a clear anatomical diagnosis. The Beverly Hills orthopedist eventually diagnosed spine "instability," but what does that mean? It sounds frightening, and certainly implies the need for something to shore up the spine.

But remember that the vertebrae have facet joints to help maintain alignment, as well as the muscles and ligaments that "shrink-wrap" the spine. So the spine doesn't easily destabilize in the usual sense of the word. But some doctors and physical therapists believe that many cases of back pain are due to abnormal motion around a disc—something that might result from a previous operation or from disc degeneration.

Yet there's no consensus on how to measure or define such instability. The term is bandied about loosely. One spine surgeon said, "Spinal instability is routinely given as a diagnosis to these patients with chronic lower-back pain. It is a term used to justify an operation. And it's a great diagnosis because it can't be directly disproved." In the absence of an obvious displacement of a vertebra, Groopman now calls it "not a real diagnosis."

So "instability" rarely means that one building block is falling off the one below, as some people might envision. Unfortunately, in the absence of a true spine deformity, it's unclear how effective a fusion really is.

And by spine deformity, I mean a severe curvature, or scoliosis; or spondylolisthesis, the type of slip that General Fridovich described. Fusion surgery has the best track record in these situations.

How successful is spine fusion surgery in the absence of these deformities? One study directly compared fusion surgery with rehabilitation for patients with ongoing back pain after an unsuccessful disc operation. This was exactly the situation Groopman faced at his second operation. Unfortunately, this study wasn't done until well after Groopman had his surgery. In this randomized trial, surgery had no advantage over rehabilitation. In fact, there was a slight trend in favor of rehabilitation.

What about fusion surgery as a first operation for degenerative discs, in the absence of the deformities noted above? Comparisons with rigorous, structured rehabilitation suggest only a small, if any, advantage for surgery. There have also been some studies comparing fusion surgery with newer surgical implants, and these offer success rates according to criteria set by the FDA.

Here's how the FDA defined a successful result from fusion surgery. The patient had to experience a substantial improvement in daily functioning; the vertebral bones had to actually fuse together; the screws and rods had to be in the right place by X-ray; the patient had to have no nerve damage from the surgery; and the patient had to go at least two years without a new operation. This doesn't seem to be asking too much.

Even so, by these criteria, the success rate of fusion surgery in one study was worse than a coin toss. Just 41 percent of fusion patients had a successful outcome. In another study, which examined a different fusion technique, the success rate was very similar: 47 percent. In this study, 80 percent of patients were still taking opioid painkillers two years after the operation. And some of the most prominent spine surgeons in the country performed these operations.

These figures contrast with widely cited success rates of 90 percent that some spine surgery centers tout on their websites. But those figures often refer simply to successful fusion of the bones, not to success as the FDA defined it. I suspect that with more rigorous criteria, these advertised rates wouldn't hold up.

In studies of patients with work-related back pain who receive workers' compensation, we might use return to work as a rough measure of success from spine fusion surgery. In these studies, far fewer than half the patients return to work within two years. The actual proportion ranges from about 26 to 36 percent.

Considering spine surgery in general, Consumer Reports surveyed almost one thousand readers who had undergone back surgery of any sort during the past five years. Only 34 percent said they were "completely satisfied" with the results. About 60 percent were "very" or "completely" satisfied. But this was much less than the percentage satisfied with hip or knee replacement surgery.

Many people imagine that after surgery their pain will be gone. But in most studies, for most patients, pain is improved but isn't cured. After a later, unrelated operation on his wrist, Dr. Groopman commented, "Frankly, I had hoped for 100 percent, and like most patients I expected to be restored to pristine condition. More often than not, that is unrealistic."

One way to estimate how many patients have serious ongoing back problems after surgery is to ask how many end up having a second back operation, as Groopman did. In large populations, this figure is almost one out of ten within two years and one out of five within ten years. And the likelihood of repeat surgery is higher after a fusion operation than after a decompression operation alone.

Over a seventeen-year time span, the number of fusion operations in the United States has soared over 600 percent. If success rates are modest, why has their popularity exploded?

Chapter 8

SURGICAL GADGETS
AND THE EXPLOSION
OF FUSION SURGERY

n 2008, Arkansas neurosurgeon Patrick Chan pleaded guilty to taking kickbacks. The case could have been made for TV. It involved the FBI, a sting operation, concealed video cameras, and cash payments. Chan faced criminal charges of taking kickbacks for agreeing to use specific spinal devices. The devices were the kinds of screws and rods that surgeons use routinely in spinal fusion surgery.

Several news accounts described the investigation of Dr. Chan. A woman representing medical device companies revealed to federal agents that she was splitting her sales commissions with Chan. Chan had suggested the arrangement, which let him collect whenever he bought or leased equipment.

The woman cooperated with the FBI to videotape the exchange of money. In one tape, "Dr. Chan is seen taking the money and putting it in his desk drawer without any questions," according to a U.S. Attorney. After Chan's arrest, a search of his car uncovered $8,000 in cash that the FBI had supplied to the sales rep to give to Chan.

This sounds bad. Indeed, a judge sentenced Chan to three years' probation and a $25,000 fine. The judge also required Chan to pay $23,000 to the FBI to cover the cost of the investigation. That may seem like a modest penalty for a neurosurgeon, but there was more to come.

At the same time as he pleaded guilty to the criminal charges, Dr. Chan agreed to pay $1.5 million to settle a civil lawsuit. The suit was filed by a whistle-blower, John Thomas of Little Rock. Thomas was a former medical device sales representative. He claimed that Chan stopped buying equipment from him when Thomas refused to offer kickbacks, even though Chan made it known that other companies were offering them.

Among other things, Thomas's suit claimed that the scheme involved "sham physician consulting contracts, bogus research studies, and expensive gifts" to Chan and other doctors. Thomas claimed that several device manufacturers were involved. In making the settlement, Chan did not admit any wrongdoing.

The manufacturers that Thomas mentioned in the suit included Blackstone Medical, a subsidiary of Orthofix International, and Synthes. These companies and several other organizations denied the allegations.

Perhaps it's no surprise that Dr. Chan and several companies also faced lawsuits from patients. Here the claim was that Chan performed unnecessary surgery so that he could receive the kickbacks. This claim hints at a new temptation. A doctor might be tempted not only to use a certain company's products but also to operate when the need was questionable.

It may be comforting to think—or hope—that Chan's story is unique, but the whistle-blower's attorney suggested otherwise. The attorney asserted, "Dr. Chan is only one piece of a big scheme that has been going on across the United States. This is by no means confined to Arkansas."

Sure enough, in 2012, Orthofix International agreed to a $32 million settlement with the U.S. government. The Justice Department argued that the company offered "kickbacks to spinal surgeons in the form of phony consulting and royalty agreements, and travel and entertainment."

The suit resulted from yet another whistle-blower, Susan Hutcheson. Hutcheson was a former regional manager with an Orthofix subsidiary. Hutcheson's allegations were colorful. She claimed that the entertainment offered to surgeons included expensive dinners, visits to strip clubs, and payment for prostitutes.

Hutcheson named Dr. Chan in her suit but also listed sixty-seven other doctors and other medical firms. The suit claimed that Orthofix paid some doctors up to $8,000 a month under phony consulting agreements. There also were bogus research grants for up to $18,000, according to the suit.

As if that weren't enough, Orthofix paid another $42 million to resolve a separate whistle-blower suit. That suit alleged kickbacks to doctors who used the company's bone growth stimulators. These devices are applied after surgery with the goal of faster healing, often in fusion operations.

That was on top of another $34 million for claims of defrauding Medicare over the bone growth stimulators. And on top of five guilty pleas by Orthofix employees to criminal charges related to kickbacks. But the hits kept coming.

Also in 2012, Orthofix agreed to pay $5 million to settle charges from the Securities and Exchange Commission. Here the claim was that Orthofix paid routine bribes, referred to as "chocolates," to Mexican government officials. The "chocolates" included cash, laptop computers, and televisions. The SEC said these were in exchange for lucrative sales contracts with government hospitals.

So Dr. Chan wasn't the only doctor involved. But you may figure that Orthofix was unusual. You would hope that Orthofix was the only company accused of kickbacks and questionable behavior. Once again, the evidence suggests otherwise.

Recall that in 2006 Medtronic agreed to pay the federal government $40 million to settle similar kickback allegations. Medtronic is the largest maker of spine implants. The Justice Department accused the company of paying surgeons through "sham consulting agreements, sham royalty agreements and lavish trips to desirable locations." The company denied any wrongdoing.

Then, in 2007, four other device manufacturers agreed to a $310 million settlement for very similar claims. Once again, the Justice Department argued that the companies were using fake consulting agreements to persuade surgeons to use their products. The then U.S. Attorney Chris Christie, now the Republican governor of New Jersey, initiated the inquiry.

The *New York Times* quoted Christie as saying, "This industry routinely violated anti-kickback statutes. . . . Prior to our investigation, many orthopedic surgeons in this country made decisions predicated on how much money they could make—choosing which device to implant by going to the highest bidder." All the companies denied any wrongdoing.

Christie's allegations had to do with knee and hip replacements, rather than spinal implants. But the same companies also make spinal implants. And these multiple settlements suggest that the kickback allegations weren't limited to exceptional cases.

The dollar amounts of these settlements sound huge to most of us. But in 2009, Medtronic had about $3.5 billion in sales. By my estimate, their $40 million settlement was about three workdays' revenue. The publisher of an orthopedic newsletter said of the $310 million settlement for joint replacements, "This is being viewed as a speeding ticket for these companies."

Kickbacks could influence which device a surgeon chooses, but they could also simply encourage the use of more devices. As the suits against Dr. Chan suggested, they may also encourage surgery in situations where the need is questionable.

Dr. Charles Rosen, an orthopedic surgeon at the University of California at Irvine, leads a doctors' organization called the Association for Medical Ethics. His observations reinforce the concern about the use of unnecessary surgical implants and surgery. Consistent with the kickback lawsuits, Rosen told a Senate committee that surgeons often receive huge consulting fees from companies in return for using their products. He also noted that the agreements encouraged promoting specific devices at medical meetings. Rosen testified, "Patients usually don't know of this conflict, which leads frequently to unnecessary implants and surgery."

The Growth of Fusion Surgery

Spinal fusion surgery has soared in this country over the last two decades. According to government statistics, surgeons performed almost 61,000 fusion operations in 1993. But in 2011, they performed 465,000 operations. That's a relative increase of 660 percent. Over those years, the U.S. population increased by just 20 percent. The average hospital charge for a spinal fusion in 2011 was $100,785.

The "national bill" for those operations in 2011 was almost $47 billion. That made spinal fusion surgery, in aggregate, the most costly type of in-hospital surgery in the United States.

Surgeons sometimes perform spinal fusion operations for serious spine deformities, like scoliosis or spondylolisthesis. Recall that spondylolisthesis is a forward slip of one vertebra over the one below. That was the reason for General David Fridovich's surgery. We noted earlier that fusion surgery has the best track record for these conditions.

Fusion surgery is also valuable in certain cases of spinal trauma, spine fractures, and cancer or infection of the vertebrae. But these are unusual circumstances and don't account for the increase in spinal fusion operations.

Instead, the most common reason for spinal fusions may also be the most controversial. And that is simply worn-out discs, or "degenerative" discs. National data suggest that this is not only the most common but also the most rapidly increasing reason for fusion operations.

As we saw from MRI scans, a third of people under age forty have degenerative discs, and nearly everyone over age sixty does. Also recall that nearly everyone gets low back pain sooner or later. Combine these circumstances, and nearly everyone becomes a potential candidate for spinal fusion surgery.

Surgery for worn-out discs is controversial because in randomized trials there appears to be little advantage over rigorous rehabilitation.

We've already noted that rates of fusion surgery vary widely around the country. We've also seen that success rates seem to run between 40 and 50 percent.

Aside from kickbacks, consulting fees, and royalties, payment levels favor spinal fusion surgery over simpler operations. In the Medicare population, a surgeon might be paid $600 to $800 for a decompression operation. But a complex fusion operation, involving multiple spinal levels, might pay ten times more.

Hospitals often benefit financially as well, and the device makers certainly do. The *Wall Street Journal* reported that pedicle screws cost less than $100 apiece to make but sell for $1,000 to $2,000 apiece.

Is there really unnecessary spinal surgery? Many surgeons think so, including Dr. Rosen. Remember that neurosurgeon Edward Benzel thought that only half the fusions performed in the United States were appropriate.

In comparing the United States with other developed countries, my colleague Dan Cherkin found that the U.S. rate of back surgery is about twice the rate in Canada, Australia, New Zealand, and most European countries. It's roughly five times the rate in England. But epidemiologic studies offer no hint that we have weaker spines or more disc problems here than in other countries.

Our research shows not only that fusion operations in the United States are increasing, but also that the complexity of the procedures is increasing. This means more discs involved, more extensive involvement of the vertebrae, and more metal implants. Dr. Rosen noted, "You can easily put $30,000 worth of hardware in a person during a fusion surgery."

More complex surgery is linked to higher complication rates. It appears to increase the need for repeat surgery as well. Yet any benefits in greater pain relief or easier daily activities remain unclear. A randomized trial comparing three types of fusion operations found that more complex operations didn't produce better pain relief or daily functioning. But the most complex surgery had the highest complication rate and the highest likelihood of ending in yet another operation.

The Continuous Stream
of New Spinal Products

A newer alternative to fusion surgery is the use of artificial discs to replace the worn-out natural discs. Following the logic of hip and knee replacement for worn-out joints, this sounds attractive. But like fusion surgery, the artificial discs are no panacea.

In fact, it's not clear whether artificial discs offer any advantage over fusion surgery in the low back. Studies of artificial discs in the low back found success rates of 53 to 57 percent by FDA criteria for success. That's awfully close to a coin toss and only slightly better than fusion. The FDA concluded that the discs were "not inferior" to a spine fusion.

The biggest unknown is how long the artificial discs will last. The hope is that they'll last a lifetime, of course. But the experience with artificial hips and knees is that some wear out. Removing a failed artificial disc is technically difficult, and the solution is often to perform a fusion operation. It's simply too soon to know how durable the artificial discs will be. And they're often being placed into people at a younger age than most hip or knee replacements.

Aside from screws and discs, device manufacturers create a steady stream of other new spine products to sell. One of these is a protein that promotes bone growth. Surgeons often use this material with the goal of enhancing the success of spinal fusion operations. There are actually several related proteins, called bone morphogenetic proteins, or BMP. The most commonly used preparation is called recombinant human BMP-2, or InFuse, made by Medtronic.

Many orthopedic surgeons saw the isolation and purification of BMP as a major advance. It meant that one needed less bone to place at the site of surgery to get two vertebrae to fuse together. It meant that successful fusion of the bones with a solid connection might be more likely.

Early studies suggested that using the protein might reduce the need for future surgery. They also reported no complications from this substance, even though it has rather complex biological properties.

Uptake of InFuse, approved in 2002, was rapid. It soon achieved almost $1 billion per year in sales for Medtronic. But the narrative of a breakthrough began to fray in 2011.

Some studies suggested that men receiving InFuse had an increased rate of retrograde ejaculation, a condition that can cause sterility. A review of FDA reports, in contrast to published research articles, uncovered other problems. The FDA reports suggested that some patients had excessive bone growth, worse postoperative pain, or other complications. Also in 2011, the FDA decided not to approve a higher-strength version of InFuse because of concerns that it might cause cancer.

Because it oversees Medicare, the Senate Finance Committee found these revelations alarming. It began to investigate the influence of the manufacturer, Medtronic, on the studies of InFuse. This was the same committee that investigated manufacturers of opioid painkillers. The investigation included a review of internal company documents and e-mails.

To make a long story short, here are some of the committee's findings, released in October 2012.

- Medtronic was heavily involved in drafting, editing, and shaping medical journal articles about InFuse. The doctors who wrote those articles received significant amounts of money through royalties and consulting fees from Medtronic.
- Medtronic paid a total of about $210 million to the doctors who wrote Infuse studies from 1996 through 2010.
- Company e-mails showed that a Medtronic employee argued against publishing all the adverse events possibly associated with Infuse.

Because of the controversy, Medtronic agreed in 2012 to provide the raw data from its studies to outside researchers. Two separate teams— one in England and one in the United States—independently analyzed the data.

Both teams concluded that there was no clinical advantage to using InFuse compared with ordinary fusion techniques. They found no differences with regard to pain, use of pain medication, or return to work. The editors who published the two reports remarked that BMP "does not improve pain or function and increases adverse events, possibly including cancer."

Both teams determined that earlier articles misrepresented the harms of BMP. The concluding line from one team was, "On the basis of the currently available evidence, it is difficult to identify clear indications for rhBMP-2 in spinal fusion."

Even critics of BMP acknowledge that there may be a place for the protein, in the most complex or high-risk fusion operations. But these situations aren't yet defined or proven, and are far less common than the widespread use of BMP.

Returning to the Senate committee report, we learn that about 85 percent of InFuse use was off-label. That meant surgeons used it in ways that weren't FDA approved. The report also tabulated Medtronic payments to the doctors who wrote the company-sponsored research studies. There were thirteen doctors who received more than $1 million each during a fifteen-year period. The individual amounts ranged from $1.7 million to $34 million, and there were additional payments to organizations owned by the same doctors.

These doctors are some of the most influential and well-known spine surgeons in the country. In the argot of the medical industry, they are key opinion leaders (KOLs), who appear at nearly every major meeting of spine surgeons. Their opinions are highly regarded.

Their comments on who should have a spinal fusion operation, how it should be performed, and what products might be used are highly influential. Other companies provide payments to key opinion leaders as well. Even though it's not advertising in the usual sense, this is part of the marketing strategy of most drug and device companies. For the companies, having key opinion leaders simply offer favorable opinions in casual conversations is marketing gold.

The device manufacturers and surgeons themselves often argue that these paid arrangements don't constitute conflicts of interest, much less kickbacks. The key opinion leaders maintain that they're not paid for using specific products, so they have no conflict of interest.

They and the companies argue that consulting fees and royalties promote collaboration between practicing surgeons and industry. This helps to refine surgical products and develop new ones to benefit patients. From this perspective, the surgeons deserve compensation for "intellectual property" that sparks innovation.

There's certainly some truth to these arguments. But the various lawsuits and criminal investigations suggest that there's a blurry line between consulting fees and kickbacks. The term "ghost patents" has crept into the vocabulary, much like ghostwriting. This suggests that a prominent individual gets credit for a company's work, justifying royalty payments.

In an investigation of payments to surgeons, for example, the *Wall Street Journal* couldn't find patents for some surgeons who received millions of dollars. A spokesperson for Medtronic argued that "intellectual property doesn't necessarily have to be patented." But a skeptic might wonder what nonpatented intellectual property is worth millions.

Like most people, surgeons, hospital executives, and corporate moguls are economically rational. Most will not pass up opportunities for income. But I don't want to leave the impression that money is the only reason for the rapid growth of spinal fusion surgery.

Many spine surgeons sincerely believe that providing more fusions is better medicine. Doctors in general share the common public perception that more is better, and more expensive is better. "You get what you pay for" is a common assumption.

Surgeons are a competitive lot and want to be on the cutting edge of new developments, so to speak. Here the assumption is that newer is better. Most are truly doing what they believe is best for their patients. But it's hard to tell how much paid key opinion leaders have influenced these perceptions.

Furthermore, surgeons like the challenge of complex surgery. Perhaps there's a macho attraction to aggressive surgery. A famous cancer surgeon once argued, "Lesser surgery is done by lesser surgeons." Medical historian Barron Lerner, himself a doctor, noted that "well-meaning cancer doctors . . . have confused doing more for patients with doing what is best for them. History tells us that this 'more is better' dictum is rarely true." This may also be the case with spine surgery.

All these factors may have contributed to the meteoric increase in spinal fusion surgery. Like some other treatments, spinal fusion has an important place but may be overused. Furthermore, these stories suggest that caution is appropriate when we consider spine surgery innovations. As some colleagues argue, "newly approved is not the same as new and improved."

If spinal fusion—or other types of spine surgery—aren't guaranteed to succeed, what about injections? Could spinal injections even stave off the need for surgery?

Chapter 9

THE POINTED
SEARCH FOR RELIEF

Injections, Ablations, and Blocks, Oh My!

President Kennedy got a variety of injections for back pain. Some were odd concoctions from "Dr. Feelgood," but others were simply local anesthetic injections provided by Dr. Janet Travell.

Travell was an advocate of trigger point injections. These are injections into muscles at places that seem particularly tender or seem to trigger pain. They usually involve injection of a local anesthetic drug or a cortisone-like drug. Or both.

Trigger point injections don't sound controversial, but later experience at the Institute of Medicine proved otherwise. The Institute of Medicine is perhaps the most prestigious group of health experts in the United States. It was chartered by Congress to formulate advice on difficult health issues. It relies on volunteer doctors and scientists to develop balanced answers to nationally important questions. In the 1980s, a panel at the Institute of Medicine prepared a report on chronic pain.

In preparing the report, Travell's close colleague, Dr. David Simons, crossed swords with other panel members. The panel couldn't even agree whether trigger points exist, much less whether injections were appropriate.

Like our Congress, the participants couldn't find much middle ground. In the end, the monograph had to include two chapters—one advocating trigger point injections and the other arguing that their very existence was controversial.

The poor consensus and bitter arguments over spinal injections continue today. Consider two clinical guideline efforts that addressed spinal injections.

In 2009, a British guideline panel completed a thorough review of research studies on treating back pain. Based on the best studies, one of the panel's recommendations was "Do not offer injections of therapeutic substances into the back for non-specific low back pain."

This conclusion was simply too much to bear for some members of the British Pain Society. And so, like the Institute of Medicine report, the guideline became a source of controversy. The British Pain Society includes many specialists who perform spinal injections. The society vented its spleen on its own president, who was an independent adviser to the guideline panel. That president was Professor Paul Watson, head of pain management and rehabilitation at the University of Leicester.

Watson has a clean-shaven thin face, balding light brown hair, and oval glasses. He sits on the editorial boards of several medical journals and is a prolific researcher. He was trained as a physical therapist and has a PhD, but he isn't a medical doctor. He was the first nonphysician president of the British Pain Society. Perhaps that made him an easy target for the physician members of the society.

And perhaps because physical therapists don't perform injections, some doctors in the society argued that Watson had a conflict of interest. That is, he might favor treatment without injections because that would steer patients to physical therapy rather than injection therapy. Watson's critics also argued that the guideline panel failed to consider some research that was more favorable to injections.

Although opinion was divided, some society members wanted Watson to repudiate the guidelines or resign as society president. When he failed to condemn the guidelines, the society voted him out of office.

Directors of the British National Institute for Health and Clinical Excellence, which sponsored the guidelines, defended Watson in a public letter. In typical British style, they didn't mince words. They said, "The society's sustained campaign against a highly respected pain management and rehabilitation expert is shameful and professional victimisation of the worst kind. . . . The British Pain Society has made its president a scapegoat because some of its members refuse to accept that there is not the scientific evidence to support their interventions. It is a sad day for the freedom of experts to express views, evidence based medicine, and the ideals of the medical profession."

On this side of the Atlantic, similar conflicts have been at work. This was dramatized by a similar guideline effort that generated similar controversy.

At the same time as the British guideline, the American Pain Society sponsored a guideline panel on injections for back pain.

This panel's conclusion was the same as the British guideline panel's. It found that there was too little evidence to recommend injections for back pain alone. It noted that one type of injection—epidural steroid injections—was moderately effective for people with sciatica. Even for sciatica, they concluded that these injections offered short-term but not long-term symptom relief. I'll explain what epidural injections are shortly.

The panel concluded that there was just too little scientific evidence to judge if several other types of injections were effective. And it recommended strongly against certain types of injections.

As with the British Pain Society, these conclusions were simply too much to bear for the American Society of Interventional Pain Physicians, or ASIPP. "Interventional procedure" is the generic name for a host of treatments that involve injecting medications or severing nerves to relieve pain. These procedures all involve needles of some description.

Doctors who specialize in these techniques call themselves interventional pain specialists, or interventionalists. Others sometimes call them "injectionists" for short. When the American Pain Society published its guideline, ASIPP responded with lengthy critiques and its own guideline. An interventionalist from Kentucky, Dr. Laxmaiah Manchikanti, led the ASIPP response. The ensuing debate came to be dubbed "Guideline Warfare."

Yet even Dr. Manchikanti acknowledged that doctors perform too many epidural steroid injections. He was quoted by the *New York Times* as saying, "We are doing too many of these, and many of those don't meet the proper criteria."

As Manchikanti's comment suggests, ongoing controversies in Britain and the United States haven't slowed explosive growth in the use of spinal injections. As one example, our analysis of Medicare data showed a 271 percent increase in epidural steroid injections between 1994 and 2001. Then, from 2000 to 2011, there was another 168 percent increase.

Why have these procedures become so popular? Several factors are probably at play, but good reimbursement seems to be one of them. Dr. Seth Waldman, who performs spinal injections at New York's Hospital for Special Surgery, says, "In medicine, if you are able to stick a needle into a person, you are reimbursed at a much better rate by the insurance company. So there is a tremendous drive to perform invasive procedures."

You may have noticed that ongoing controversies regarding pain treatments seem to be the norm. Debates over the proper roles of opioids and surgery, for example, are just as vigorous as the debates over injections. This should be a hint that there are no slam-dunk treatments in the pain world, though advocates of each treatment would have you believe otherwise.

Let's look a bit closer at the range of needling treatments. Just as there are many varieties of back operations, there are many varieties of spinal injections. After explaining what they are, let's examine some of the scientific evidence about their efficacy. Finally, we'll look at some possible downsides of these treatments.

Kennedy's doctor, Janet Travell, advocated trigger point injections. With these injections into the muscles, a local anesthetic temporarily blocks pain perception. If the injection includes a cortisone-like drug, that can block inflammation. This means it reduces the swelling, redness, and heat that often cause pain, though these may all be internal and invisible.

Doctors often refer to cortisone-like drugs simply as "steroids," though the term is ambiguous. For example, you also hear about athletes abusing steroids, but that refers to drugs like testosterone. Both cortisone and testosterone belong to a class of naturally occurring chemical compounds called steroids, but they have different effects.

The drugs that doctors inject for pain are usually synthetic derivatives of cortisone, and usually more potent. For our purposes, just remember that when we refer to "steroid injections," we mean these cortisone-like drugs.

The injections most often performed in pain clinics are epidural steroid injections. Rather than injections into muscles, these are injections into the spinal canal. This is the canal formed by "holes" in the vertebrae. The spinal cord runs through the spinal canal, and a tough membrane called the dura surrounds it. The target of an epidural steroid injection is the space inside the bony canal but outside the dura—hence the term epidural. This is the same space where some women get epidural anesthetics for pain relief during childbirth.

There are several variations in technique for performing epidural steroid injections. Experts argue over which steroid drug is best, what volume of the liquid drug they should use, what the best approach with the needle is, and whether they need fluoroscopy (video X-ray) to check the placement of the needle. Opinions are strong, but the evidence on these details is weak.

Doctors most often perform epidural steroid injections when there's a herniated disc pressing on a nerve. The pressure often causes inflammation of the nerve, which in turn gives rise to the pain of sciatica. The goal is to inject the steroid as close to the inflamed nerve as possible.

Another popular type of injection is into the facet joints. The facets are small joints toward the back of each vertebra. There's a pair of these joints—left and right—between each pair of vertebrae, and they help to maintain proper alignment of the spine while allowing flexibility. Though they're small, like finger joints, they can develop arthritis just like joints anywhere else in the body.

Two types of facet joint treatments have become popular. One is injection of a steroid into the joint, again with the rationale of reducing inflammation. The other is called a medial branch nerve block.

The medial branch nerves are small nerves that come from the facet joints and transmit pain signals from them. In a typical medial branch nerve block, a doctor first injects local anesthetic around this nerve. If that injection—and sometimes a second injection—provides pain relief, it's followed by a radiofrequency neurotomy, which uses heat to sever the nerve and interrupt pain signals. It's also sometimes called "denervation." Although the nerve may eventually regrow, doctors intend a neurotomy to provide relief for a year or more.

There are several other injection or neurotomy types, in other locations. But they generally use techniques much like the epidural or facet joint injections.

What's the evidence that these things work? And how compelling is that evidence?

Several expert groups have tried to compile the relevant research studies. Some come from multidisciplinary doctor panels, which include pain experts who don't directly benefit from doing injections. Organizations like the Institute of Medicine prefer such panels, arguing that input from multiple perspectives helps to reduce any bias. Dr. Roger Chou, a colleague at Oregon Health and Science University, led one of the most rigorous reviews.

Dr. Chou sports a mustache and short goatee and has thick black hair. He's average height and thin, as you'd expect from someone who runs a marathon—or two—every month. He's a primary care doctor rather than a pain specialist.

Chou heads a center at our medical school that receives funding from the federal Agency for Healthcare Research and Quality. His center routinely conducts meticulous research reviews on a wide variety of topics. The center has sophisticated strategies for searching the research literature and for grading the quality of the studies.

Dr. Chou led the American Pain Society's guideline effort on spinal injections. That guideline panel had twenty-three expert members and three advisers. The group represented a wide variety of medical specialties, including doctors who routinely perform spinal injections.

For trigger point injections, the panel concluded that there was simply too little research to know whether they work. The studies the panel found were too few, too small, too poor in quality, and too variable in terms of patients and injection techniques.

The panel recommended against steroid injections into the facet joints. There were consistent findings among high-quality studies indicating that the results of these injections were no better than sham therapy.

The panel also recommended against some other types of injection for low back pain. These included prolotherapy, in which a doctor injects an irritant solution into ligaments. The theory is that the resulting inflammation will "tighten" the ligaments and reduce painful motion.

The Pain Society also recommended against injection of steroids into the discs of the spine. The group found too little data to recommend for or against Botox injections to relax spinal muscles. Similarly, they found too little to recommend for or against sacroiliac joint injections.

What about injecting local anesthetic into the facets, followed by radiofrequency neurotomy of the medial branch nerve? After considering the highest-quality studies, the panel concluded that there was too little evidence to make a recommendation for or against the technique.

What about epidural steroid injections? These are the most common injections provided by interventional pain specialists.

Here the panel's conclusions were mixed. For low back pain without sciatica or for people with spinal stenosis—a narrowing of the spinal canal—panel members concluded there were too few data to make a recommendation.

But for patients with sciatica from a herniated disc, they recommended that doctors discuss epidural injection as an option. That discussion, they said, should describe the inconsistent results from research studies. And it should note that there seem to be "moderate short-term benefits and lack of long-term benefits."

Advocates often argue that epidural steroid injections could prevent the need for disc surgery in some patients. Some of the randomized trials of epidural injections followed patients to see if those who received steroids had less subsequent surgery than those who got placebo injections. Unfortunately, most of these studies failed to show a reduction in subsequent surgery.

Furthermore, injection rates vary among small geographic areas just as surgery rates do. When we examined these geographic variations, we found that where there were more injections, there also were more operations. I don't think injections were *causing* more surgery. But different regions evolve more or less aggressive treatment styles. I suspect that an aggressive injection style and an aggressive surgery style go together. It certainly didn't seem that more injections were leading to *less* surgery.

Like the American Pain Society, the American Academy of Neurology concluded that epidural injections might offer short-term relief for people with sciatica. And that's important for some patients. But the neurologists concluded that the injections wouldn't decrease the need for surgery, improve daily function, or relieve pain beyond three months.

The Pain Society conclusions drove some interventionalists crazy. Led by Dr. Manchikanti, members of the interventionalist group, ASIPP, prepared a lengthy rebuttal to the Pain Society guidelines and developed their own set of guidelines. These were published in their own medical journal. They also were developed entirely by doctors who perform the injections rather than by a multidisciplinary panel with fewer vested interests.

Authors of the Pain Society guidelines subsequently pointed to erroneous statements and inadequate scientific methods in the ASIPP responses, but both groups defended their positions.

What did independent doctors and scientists have to say? By and large, independent reviews have been in line with the American Pain Society's interpretation of the research literature. An independent review of ten international guidelines gave the Pain Society's guideline on injections the only perfect score on criteria related to "rigor of development." Another review of the studies on injection suggested, "Overall, there is only low to very low quality evidence to support the use of injection therapy and denervation procedures over placebo or other treatments for patients with chronic low back pain." A more recent commentary concluded that "given the weak scientific evidence base and the availability of noninvasive and more effective alternatives, physicians and policy makers should not recommend the use of injection therapy for patients with low back pain and sciatica."

And of course, as we saw, the British guideline panel independently reached very similar conclusions.

What about side effects? Happily, major side effects of these injections are rare. They can include allergic reactions, bleeding, and infection. Very rarely, they can cause nerve or spinal cord injury.

But the exploding rate of injections magnifies the risks. And recent events remind us that the side effects, though rare, can't be ignored.

In September 2012, Tennessee public health officials reported the first cases of fungal meningitis associated with a contaminated steroid solution. The steroid preparation was being used for epidural injections.

Despite a recall of the contaminated solution, made by the New England Compounding Center, incubating infections emerged over several months. By July 2013, the U.S. Centers for Disease Control reported 749 cases and 61 deaths related to these infections. They were reported from twenty states. Some of the patients who didn't die had strokes or signs of serious spinal cord injury.

This wasn't the first time that contaminated drugs caused a problem. A similar but smaller outbreak of fungal meningitis related to epidural steroid injections occurred in 2002.

Furthermore, there's growing concern about complications related to systemwide effects of the steroid drugs. After doctors inject them, the steroids spread and the bloodstream ultimately absorbs them. Then they can have effects throughout the body. These effects include a litany of the same side effects that steroids can cause if they're taken by mouth.

One of these side effects is osteoporosis. A recent study of postmenopausal women found that after even a single epidural steroid injection, there was a measurable decrease in bone density in the hip. Along with this, there appeared to be an increased risk of vertebral fractures. Other doctors have noticed increases in blood sugar, another well-known consequence of these drugs.

In the end, there are a host of unanswered questions about the effectiveness of spinal injections, and we're just learning about some of the risks. Some types of injections clearly appear to be ineffective. For others, legitimate controversy remains.

In a situation where there are definite complications and uncertain benefits, caution is appropriate. This is an area of medicine where there are few "right" answers. Patients should insist on learning their options, studying the benefits and risks, taking an active role in making decisions, and having their eyes wide open with regard to the uncertainties.

If injections are only modestly effective at best, why do some people seem so much better after an injection?

Chapter 10

WHY WOULD YOU GET BETTER AFTER USELESS THERAPY?

I've been hard on some widely accepted and popular treatments for back pain. At this point, some readers have to be thinking, "This guy doesn't know what he's talking about. I got Treatment X, which he claims is useless, and I got better. It obviously works."

Treatment X might be bed rest, TENS therapy, Neurontin tablets, facet injections, fusion surgery for degenerative discs, or some other treatment whose benefits I've minimized. How could someone get better if these things are ineffective?

First, we might start with a well-known fallacy often cited by lawyers: *post hoc, ergo propter hoc*. Lawyers are almost as fond of Latin as doctors are. This phrase, roughly translated, means that if one event followed another, the first event must have caused the second. The error in this thinking is probably obvious to all of us when we think about daily life.

If I put on a new blue shirt today, and the Seahawks win, it's probably not because I put on the new blue shirt. But if it happens at the next game, I might think, "Every time I wear the blue shirt, the Seahawks win!" This is how superstitions get started.

There's a great temptation with medical treatments to assume that if we got better after a treatment, it was because of the treatment. The classic example that vexes doctors is the patient requesting antibiotics for a cold. "I got antibiotics last time and got better fast," the patient says. In doing so, he fails to recognize that this is what colds tend to do anyway, and that cold viruses eat antibiotics for breakfast.

Maybe it seemed like that last cold was longer than usual and got better quickly after the antibiotics. But the drawn-out course likely just meant that the patient was closer to having it improve on its own. The *post hoc* fallacy is especially seductive when symptoms have lasted a long time.

Several years ago, my wife, Lynda, and I chuckled at the way this fallacy might easily have duped us. She didn't have back pain, but she had another painful musculoskeletal problem that baffles doctors: a frozen shoulder. This occurs when tissues surrounding the shoulder joint seem to tighten, for unknown reasons. It's as if the muscles and ligaments shrink-wrap the joint so tightly that it hurts and can barely move.

Against all odds, Lynda and her three siblings are all redheads, despite their brunette parents. Lynda sometimes refers to them as the Farkel family, recalling the loony family of redheaded kids who were regulars on *Rowan and Martin's Laugh-In*. In addition, the siblings were all very athletic. Lynda and her brothers often shared the winner's circle at school track meets. To this day, Lynda can run circles around me on a bicycle, a 5K run, or a tennis court. So it was unusual for her to face physical limitations.

Lynda could barely sleep because the shoulder was so painful. At a parking lot that dispensed parking tickets, she had to get out of the car to pull the ticket because she couldn't raise her shoulder. Putting carry-on bags in the overhead bin of an airplane was out of the question. She saw an orthopedic surgeon and a physical therapist but was skeptical that either would be very helpful. This went on for a year without relief.

One day, Lynda finally wondered aloud if she should try acupuncture. I told her it couldn't hurt and might be worth a try. Like many busy people, though, she hemmed and hawed and procrastinated making an appointment. She had reached a point of deciding she would just have to adjust and cope with the situation.

But while she procrastinated, something amazing happened. Her shoulder began to improve rapidly. On almost a daily basis, her pain was better and her motion was improving. In less than two weeks, her symptoms were almost gone. Within a month or two, she was completely back to normal, with no pain or limitations of any sort.

In retrospect, we laughed that if she had gotten acupuncture when she first mentioned it, we would now both be absolutely convinced that the acupuncture had cured her shoulder. After a year with no improvement, what else could we conclude? *Post hoc, ergo propter hoc.*

And yet what happened was actually just a natural healing process. It turns out that improvement after about a year often happens with frozen shoulders. It's what doctors call the "natural history" of the disease.

This was no placebo effect. There was no placebo. This was just the natural healing process, delayed.

With acute back pain—simply meaning back pain of recent onset—the natural history is to improve quickly. If you have acute back pain, please buy this book *immediately* so I can have the sale before you get better!

Years ago, NBA basketball star Isaiah Thomas injured his back in a fall during a playoff game against the Los Angeles Lakers. Newspaper reports indicated that Thomas soaked his body and used heat treatments for two days but "still felt too stiff to get out of bed and make it to a Detroit Pistons practice."

Nonetheless, by the next day, not only could he move around, he was able to play professional basketball in a highly competitive playoff game, giving the Pistons "an unexpected spark," according to news accounts. The Pistons won that return game, although they lost the series in game seven.

We have to figure that Thomas was in a world of hurt. It's unimaginable that the team's star was malingering during the NBA finals. But just two days later, he led his team to a win in a bruising sport.

We may not all recover as quickly as a professional athlete or get the same loving attention from a cadre of trainers and doctors. But even for the rest of us, acute back pain tends to improve fast.

In a pair of studies almost ten years apart, French doctor Joël Coste and his colleagues studied patients who came to the doctor for a new episode of back pain within three days of the start of the pain. They didn't consider patients with sciatica, cancer, or fractures that could explain their pain, or anyone with an episode of back pain during the previous three months.

Among these people with very recent onset of pain, almost 90 percent recovered within two to four weeks. In fact, half of them recovered in eight days. For all we know, many other people with back pain of just three days never bothered to go to a doctor and got better on their own.

Even in studies that included people with a longer duration of pain, rapid improvement over a month was normal. Even people who had to miss work because of their back pain did well. About 80 percent returned to work within a month.

Consider these expert pronouncements compiled by a skeptical physical therapist, Julie Zimmerman:

- "Mobilization and manipulation studies claim an 80 percent success rate."
- "80 percent of low back pain patients get immediate relief with epidural blocks."
- "With microcurrent therapy . . . 82 percent were pain free within 10 treatments."
- "Radiofrequency facet denervation is more than 70 percent effective."
- "In the YMCA's exercise program, 80 percent improve."
- "70–80 percent of those carefully screened for radicular symptoms benefit from surgery."

See a pattern? It looks like 70 to 80 percent of people with back pain get better no matter what you do! I think all these experts are accurately describing what they see. It's just that what they're seeing looks suspiciously like natural healing rather than actual treatment effects.

This may explain one of my favorite supermarket tabloids, whose headline blared that WD-40 cures back pain! I'll bet that it "works" 80 percent of the time. Ben Franklin described the situation aptly: "God heals, and the doctor takes the fees."

Of course, everything is not quite as rosy as this sounds. The downside of this glowing outlook is that many people get repeat episodes of pain. I've come to think of back pain as being a bit like asthma. That is, it's often a persistent condition that causes only minor problems most of the time but flares up intermittently to drive you crazy.

But the point I want to make here is that the natural healing process can fool any of us into thinking a treatment is more effective than it really is. What else might fool us?

Statisticians remind us of another problem, which they label "regression to the mean." Like all academics, they use unnecessarily complex language. What this really means is "returning to the average."

We often think of chronic conditions as constant and unchanging. But the key concept here is that even chronic, persistent symptoms wax and wane. You might have pain every day, but there are good days and bad days. The pain isn't the same all the time, even if it's chronic. It fluctuates in a seemingly random way.

But when are you most likely to seek out your doctor for help? It's not on the good days! It's on the bad days. On the days that aren't typical but are worse than average.

Now if those fluctuations in pain are more or less random, what happens next? Over time, just by chance, the fluctuations return to their average level. Regression to the mean.

This is different from the process of natural healing. Healing is a genuine physiologic process that the body carries out. The body repairs injured tissues and clears the cells and chemicals that cause inflammation and pain. Regression to the mean is just a statistical probability—that extreme symptoms are likely to return to their average level over time.

In other words, a betting man could make good money betting that most people with back pain will be somewhat improved by two to four weeks after they see a doctor. The odds are in his favor even if treatment doesn't work at all.

And that brings us to a third reason why pain might get better after useless treatment. This is one that most people immediately consider but often dismiss: the placebo effect.

A placebo is something that is designed to simulate medical therapy but has no real treatment effect. A sugar pill, for example, might be used to simulate a real pain pill. Recall that I earlier described a study in which we used a sham electrical stimulation device to simulate the real thing. A placebo injection might make use of saline solution to simulate an injection of local anesthetic or steroid.

To simulate a minor surgical procedure, doctors have even taken patients to the operating room, made a small incision in the skin, and used fake fluoroscopy to create the appearance of a real operation. They did this with patients' consent, so patients would realize they might not have a real operation.

Placebos probably don't work to save lives or affect blood tests, but studies confirm that they have important effects on pain. Even with real treatments, placebo effects can enhance the benefits.

You may figure that only gullible or weak-minded people are susceptible to placebo effects, but the reality is that we all are. Rates of placebo responses vary among studies. But in some studies, 85 percent of subjects experience placebo effects. Despite being well educated, trained in medicine, and scientifically minded, medical students respond to placebos just like everyone else.

And placebos have some surprising properties that mimic real therapy. For example, taking two pills has a better effect than taking just one. In a recent study, a more expensive placebo worked better than a less expensive one. Placebos are also associated with side effects, such as drowsiness, headaches, or nausea.

It may be that the placebo effects of physical treatments—like fake acupuncture—are stronger than the placebo effects of pills.

And surgery seems to have important placebo effects as well. In the 1950s, a popular minor operation for patients with chest pain due to heart disease (angina) was compared with a sham operation. Patients receiving the sham operation got just a small skin incision. More than half the patients who got the sham operation had significant improvement in chest pain, and over 40 percent cut down on their medication.

What about back surgery? As far as I know, no one has done a study with a sham back operation. But back in the 1970s, before we had modern imaging techniques, a Swedish surgeon reported on the outcomes of surgery among patients with back and leg pain who got a mistaken diagnosis of a herniated disc. These were people who turned out *not* to have a herniated disc when they were actually "opened up." In this situation, the surgeon simply closed the surgical incision. About 40 percent of these patients had complete relief of their back or leg pain, even though they essentially had a sham operation.

Just as an aside, that 40 percent success rate looks awfully close to the success rate of fusion surgery for degenerated discs. We noted earlier that by the FDA criteria, 41 to 47 percent of those fusion operations were successful. We might reasonably wonder if this is much more effective than a sham operation.

How do placebos work? I won't go into detail here, and there's still a lot to learn. One factor seems to be the important effect of expectations. If you expect that treatment is going to reduce your pain, that alone may reduce anxiety, fear, and the severity of pain. Things may seem more controllable, and you may be more likely to notice small improvements and to dismiss negative events.

A related factor may be a learning effect, in which any treatment comes to be associated with successful past treatments. Even favorable interactions with a doctor in the past may be enough to elicit a learned response.

Some researchers have suggested that placebo effects may result from the release of naturally occurring endorphins in the body. These substances mimic opioids in their effect on the brain and spinal cord.

But there have been conflicting results in research studies, and the role of endorphins is still unclear.

So placebo effects are important in pain treatment. Pills, injections, and surgery all cause placebo effects, and nearly everyone seems to have placebo responses. These effects accompany both fake and real treatments. Thus, we might see them with popular treatments that are ineffective as well as those that actually have a specific treatment effect.

Now we have a trio of factors that can make people get better even with ineffective therapy: natural history, regression to the mean, and placebo effects. And beyond these, other things can affect improvement in pain. A doctor's warmth, friendliness, interest, empathy, and prestige may all enhance the effects of placebos or ineffective therapy.

For example, the benefits of greater attention were apparent in studies of antidepressant drugs. Among forty-one studies, those with more frequent follow-up visits proved to have greater placebo effects. In fact, researchers found the apparent benefit of more visits in both treatment arms of these studies. That is, even in the study groups that got real antidepressant medication, more visits were linked to better outcomes.

In a study of acupuncture—for bowel problems rather than back pain—researchers compared three groups. The researchers randomly assigned one group to receive no treatment and to go on a waiting list. The second group got placebo acupuncture with very limited interaction with the therapist. And the third group got placebo acupuncture with a practitioner who displayed warmth, attention, and confidence.

Sure enough, placebo acupuncture did significantly better than no treatment by several measures. But placebo acupuncture with ample attention did significantly better than placebo acupuncture alone. In the waiting group, 28 percent reported adequate symptom relief, compared with 44 percent with placebo acupuncture alone. But in the group with both placebo acupuncture and attention, 62 percent reported adequate relief.

So now we have four factors, a foursome, that might exaggerate the real effectiveness of therapy.

This combination of factors—natural history, regression to the mean, placebo effects, and caring attention—has helped to create a legacy of useless treatments for back pain. Research has now thoroughly discredited many formerly standard treatments. Think of bed rest, traction, corsets, and plaster jackets. We can safely assume that the foursome of exaggerating factors explained their popularity.

Keep these four factors in mind every time you hear about a new "breakthrough" for treating back pain. In many cases, the benefits may be more closely related to these factors than to any specific benefit of the new treatment.

How can we figure out if any improvement from treatment is *better* than the combination of natural history, regression to the mean, placebo effects, and a caring doctor's attention? That's the magic of a comparison group, or control group, that gets a placebo. The control group experiences all these effects—just not the effect of receiving the active treatment. Now we can see if people getting the real treatment have more improvement than people who just get the foursome.

A randomized trial is simply one in which appropriate patients are assigned to real treatment or sham treatment by chance alone. This strategy generally ensures that the two groups will be as similar as possible, even in ways we can't measure. So how does the combination of natural history, regression to the mean, placebo effects, and caring attention play out in such a research study?

Earlier I described our study of transcutaneous electrical nerve stimulation, or TENS, which suggested that the treatment was ineffective. But notice, I didn't say that no one got better after TENS therapy.

In fact, the patients who got real TENS units reported, on average, a 47 percent improvement in their pain and nearly a 50 percent improvement in physical function. Those are big improvements for people who had, on average, more than four years of chronic back pain. How can we say TENS didn't work?

Because in the sham TENS group, with very similar characteristics, the patients had on average a 42 percent improvement in pain and nearly a 50 percent improvement in physical function. In other words, virtually the same results.

You can see how easy it would be to make wrong judgments about treatment effectiveness based on clinical experience alone. If I were a therapist who offered TENS treatment and saw patients with long-standing back pain routinely improving by 50 percent, it would be natural for me to assume that TENS really works. But our study suggested that I might just be seeing the effects of natural history, regression to the mean, placebo effects, and empathetic attention. Those are all good things, to be sure, but not the same as real treatment effectiveness.

Another example came from our study of bed rest for back pain. Recall that we randomly assigned patients in that study to rest in bed for either two days or seven days. After three weeks of follow-up, the group assigned to a full week of bed rest had an average 35 percent improvement in physical function. Not bad! No wonder bed rest was a popular treatment for so many years.

But the group assigned to just two days of bed rest had a 36 percent improvement in physical function—essentially the same. And these patients missed less work. That foursome of nonspecific factors seemed to be at play. Suddenly, a week of bed rest didn't look so attractive.

All these stories help explain why you might get better after useless therapy. They also help explain why doctors are fond of randomized trials with a placebo comparison group. We've already seen that many popular medical treatments don't stack up so well when we consider well-designed randomized trials.

Armed with these tools, let's examine another controversy. What about "alternative" treatments? How well do treatments like chiropractic care, acupuncture, and massage work?

Chapter 11

MANIPULATING THE PAIN

Chiropractic and Other
"Alternative" Treatments

It's no secret that medical doctors and chiropractors historically had little use for each other. Doctors often called chiropractors quacks. Chiropractors called a medical editor a medical Mussolini.

The tensions arose in part from the colorful but nonscientific origins of chiropractic care. The founder, D. D. Palmer, was a magnetic healer practicing in the Midwest in the late 1800s. He claimed that he once cured a janitor's deafness by manipulating his neck. Thus began the concept of spinal manipulation. The name "chiropractic" derives from the Greek *cheiro* (hand) and *practos* (doing by). Palmer came to believe that 95 percent of all diseases arose from misaligned or "subluxated" vertebrae.

Given this belief, Palmer and other chiropractic leaders rejected the germ theory. They attributed even diseases like smallpox to spinal subluxation. Most chiropractors rejected vaccines and antibiotics, along with other drugs, as poisons. This created a grudge between chiropractors and medical doctors.

Despite opposition to drug therapy, some chiropractors promoted homeopathic remedies and dietary supplements of unproven benefit. Such prescribing habits became another bone of contention with the medical profession.

Rancor between chiropractors and medical doctors peaked in the 1960s. This was when the American Medical Association (AMA) formed a Committee on Quackery, which was devoted to destroying the chiropractic profession. Among other things, the committee deemed it unethical for medical doctors to associate professionally with chiropractors.

Subsequent lawsuits, retractions, and evolving attitudes have softened this face-off, though ample mistrust persists on both sides. Nonetheless, some practices now have chiropractors and medical doctors working side by side. Détente is the order of the day.

Some chiropractors claim to treat a wide variety of diseases, including chronic conditions like heart failure and diabetes. But let's avoid a dispute about such claims. We'll focus just on spinal manipulation for back pain, which remains the bread and butter of chiropractic practice.

Spinal manipulation is the core treatment that all chiropractors use, though they prefer the term spinal "adjustment." There are many techniques, varying in the force delivered and the amplitude of movement.

It's unclear how spinal manipulation works to relieve pain. Various theories focus on the small facet joints in the spine, on repositioning disc material, on reducing muscle tension or stiffness, and on other possibilities. Chiropractors also often recommend therapeutic exercise and sometimes make use of massage and acupressure in addition to spinal manipulation.

Chiropractors don't have a monopoly on spinal manipulation, of course. Some osteopathic doctors perform spinal manipulation, as do some physical therapists. These groups often butt heads with each other and with state regulators regarding who can be licensed to practice spinal manipulation.

As an aside, osteopathy also originated in the late 1800s, founded by Andrew Taylor Still. Still studied as a medical doctor but was dissatisfied with treatments of the day. Given that his experience preceded sanitary practices and modern medications, his skepticism is understandable.

Still evolved a theory that musculoskeletal problems underlay most diseases and that manipulating bones and joints was a key treatment. This approach also had the advantage of avoiding the toxic effects of many of the drug remedies of the time. Just as Palmer founded the first school of chiropractic, Still founded the first school of osteopathy. Osteopathic philosophy and training, which result in a DO degree, moved closer to mainstream medicine in the twentieth century. Today, despite some past contests with the AMA reminiscent of the chiropractic story, doctors with an MD or a DO degree are strikingly similar in their practices. Perhaps the main difference is that some osteopathic doctors still offer spinal manipulation.

The public speaks with its feet and demonstrates growing acceptance of spinal manipulation. When *Consumer Reports* magazine surveyed subscribers with low back pain—fourteen thousand of them—the most popular treatment was chiropractic care. Almost 60 percent of those who saw a chiropractor were highly satisfied, compared with just 34 percent who saw a primary care medical doctor. Incidentally, physical therapists were close behind the chiropractors.

But patient satisfaction can reflect many things besides treatment effectiveness. And we've seen how anecdotal observations can be misleading. What can we learn from randomized trials of spinal manipulation?

The truth is that interpreting research studies on spinal manipulation is an exercise in frustration. And this is true for other types of complementary and alternative medicine (CAM)—like acupuncture and massage—as well.

In part, this is because advocates or detractors spin small treatment effects differently. That is, they either are or aren't enough to matter to typical patients. The comparison treatments and patient selection methods differ from study to study. Some studies try to control for placebo effects; others simply compare CAM treatments with conventional medical care. Trials have often reached differing conclusions: CAM treatments work or they don't. You can find randomized trials to support any position you choose.

Placebo effects may be an important component of CAM thera-pies. Of course, this is true of conventional medical treatments as well. Experts disagree on whether it's wise to knowingly take advantage of placebo effects in routine care.

Finally, an unspoken problem for these studies concerns the peo-ple who volunteer for them. Most volunteers probably believe they'll benefit from the CAM treatments and are favorably disposed toward them. Furthermore, they might be disappointed if they're assigned *not* to receive the CAM therapy under study. The disappointment alone might color their self-perceptions of improvement. If these things are true, we can't really tell what the results might be among people who are less favorably disposed.

So let's specify a few things before we even look at the research studies. First, we're not going to reach a definitive conclusion. Sec-ond, we're going to see that there's no slam-dunk treatment that works for everyone. On average, treatment effects are modest, at best, or we'd see a better consensus about their benefits. Of course, that's true for most conventional medical treatments as well. Third, we're likely to disagree on at least some of the conclusions, based on our personal experiences and preconceptions. But opposing camps can be civil about it.

Let's start with spinal manipulation and Dr. Dan Cherkin of Seat-tle. Dr. Cherkin has a long-standing interest in doctor-patient relation-ships and the nature of the healing process. This led him to an abiding interest in studying CAM therapy and its potential for helping patients with complex problems like back pain.

Cherkin is an outgoing man with a quick smile and an easygoing sense of humor. He has a PhD in epidemiology, the discipline that champions advances in clinical research design. He's not a medical doctor, chiropractor, physical therapist, or osteopath, so he's not an ad-vocate for any particular form of therapy.

Fifteen years ago, I worked with Dr. Cherkin and his colleagues at Group Health Cooperative in Seattle to compare chiropractic care with competing approaches. We studied more than three hundred patients with back pain, who we randomly assigned to treatment by a chiropractor, a physical therapist, or their usual primary care doctor.

A quick summary is that we found no difference between chiropractic care and physical therapy. Both were modestly better than routine care from a primary care doctor along with an educational booklet.

Several other randomized trials have compared chiropractic care with routine medical care. Unfortunately, the studies have used different measures of success, timing of follow-up, and types of comparison groups. As a result, efforts to review all the available studies conclude that the evidence on spinal manipulation is weak.

These randomized trials generally report that *on average*, spinal adjustment is no more effective than routine medical care. But also no less effective. And remember that averages result from combining big effects and small effects, along with middling effects. So examining only averages can obscure the possibility that some people had excellent results.

I've had patients who swore by chiropractors, and patients who swore at them. I've also had patients who swore by me and some who swore at me. Some patients who fail conventional medical care do well with spinal adjustment and vice versa. My conclusion is that compared with conventional medical care, spinal adjustment may be no more and no less effective, but it is *differently* effective. That is, the mechanism is different, and it seems likely that different people benefit from different treatments.

Like chiropractic adjustment, osteopathic adjustment appears to offer modest benefits in randomized trials. There's little evidence directly comparing treatment by chiropractors with treatment by osteopathic doctors.

An advantage of spinal manipulation is relative safety. In the low back, one credible estimate is that serious complications occur at about one per hundred million visits. If only the drugs I've prescribed were so safe! In the neck, serious complications are probably more common, but they're still rare.

Acupuncture is another increasingly popular CAM treatment. Its origins stretch back to ancient China. The traditional belief was that therapists should place needles at specific acupuncture points. Manipulating needles at these locations would correct the flow of *qi* (pronounced "chee"), or life energy, through channels called meridians. You may have seen ancient depictions of the meridians drawn on human figures.

An important controversy in acupuncture research has been the definition of a placebo group. There's debate, for example, about whether deliberately misplaced needling—not at acupuncture points—could have a genuine treatment effect. Or whether stimulation without puncturing the skin might also have genuine treatment effects.

For example, we've used toothpicks in some research projects, simply placing them in the same guide tubes used for real acupuncture needles. In a lead-up to one of our projects, I subjected myself to treatment with real needles or toothpicks, blinded to which was which. I was completely fooled and unable to tell the difference. I wasn't the only one; this was true for most people we tested.

With Dan Cherkin and his colleague Karen Sherman taking the lead, we designed a study similar to our chiropractic study. We compared real acupuncture, fake acupuncture, and "usual care" from a primary doctor. In this case, we assigned more than six hundred patients to the different treatment groups. The real acupuncture and the fake acupuncture groups had nearly identical results, and both were somewhat better than usual care. Use of pain medicines decreased in both the real and the fake acupuncture groups.

What do we make of this? One interpretation would be that the effects of acupuncture are entirely placebo effects, since fake acupuncture was as good as the real thing. Another interpretation would be that acupuncture really works, but the location of the needles and penetrating the skin are irrelevant. Perhaps just stimulating the skin is all that's needed.

Well-designed studies from Germany, some using misplaced needling, reported results similar to ours. Together the research studies argue against the Chinese meridian concept, or even the need for penetrating the skin. But maybe stimulating the skin works even if meridians and skin penetration are irrelevant.

Finally, a recent study combined data from individual patients who took part in twenty-nine randomized trials of acupuncture. These involved people with a variety of pain conditions, including back pain. The combined analysis concluded that real acupuncture was more effective than fake acupuncture and better than non-acupuncture treatments.

Is there any research to suggest that either fake or real acupuncture has physiological effects? Functional MRI studies and hormone measurements suggest that even superficial stimulation has some effects on the brain and endocrine systems. Other brain imaging studies suggest that true acupuncture has effects on the brain that are different from those of sham acupuncture, even if the two provide similar pain relief.

We're not going to resolve the disparate interpretations of the research results here. But it does seem that some people get significant benefit from acupuncture, whatever the mechanism. And it seems fair to conclude again that it's effective in a *different* way than conventional medical care.

Like spinal manipulation, acupuncture is remarkably safe. Serious complications are rare but can result from inserting needles too deep. In an era of disposable acupuncture needles, infections are almost nonexistent. Surveys suggest that serious complications occur less than once per hundred thousand sessions of acupuncture.

Massage is the third widely used type of CAM therapy for back pain but the least well studied. Again, it's not crystal clear why massage might work. It may have beneficial effects on the muscles and soft tissues of the back or it may just have a general relaxing effect. As with other CAM treatments, it could be that the effects result from a relaxing environment, being touched, and having a caring therapist.

Once again, Drs. Cherkin, Sherman, colleagues at Group Health, and I teamed up to do some randomized trials. This time, we assigned 401 patients with back pain to receive massage therapy or continued "usual care" from their primary doctors. We tested two types of massage, but their results were the same, so we can just refer to those together as the massage group.

The results were strikingly similar to those we saw for spinal manipulation and for acupuncture. The massage group had better outcomes than did patients in the usual care group, but the differences were modest. A small number of other randomized trials report generally similar results.

The American College of Physicians and the American Pain Society jointly developed guidelines for back pain that addressed these CAM therapies just as they addressed spinal injections. These guidelines judged spinal manipulation, acupuncture, and massage all to have benefits for patients with persistent back pain.

Another systematic review came to similar conclusions but noted that the benefit of CAM treatments appeared to be short-lived. These treatments are supplied by a health care provider, and the patient has a passive role. They may have less durable effects than treatments that engage patients more actively, such as exercise and cognitive-behavioral therapy. These are treatments we'll examine later in more detail.

The editors of *Consumer Reports* summarized their survey by noting that respondents generally rated hands-on treatments as very helpful. That included chiropractic treatments, massage, and physical therapy, as well as acupuncture. They concluded that the results were a testament to the healing power of touch, which may be a unifying factor among these treatments.

Practitioners of these "alternative" therapies sometimes feel that they're struggling for credibility in a hostile medical world. But what if patients feel like they themselves are struggling for credibility?

Chapter 12

NOBODY TAKES IT SERIOUSLY!

If you break a leg, you'll wear a cast. People will sign it, write funny things, be sympathetic, and understand why you're a little slower than usual. If you have an appendectomy, people will visit you in the hospital, they'll look at your scar, they'll ask for weeks how you're doing, and they'll understand why you're a little slower than usual. But if you have back pain, look out!

Nobody can see it. You probably won't land in the hospital. You won't have a cast or a scar. If you're limping, people may assume you're exaggerating. And if you're a little slower than usual, don't expect much sympathy or understanding. It's an invisible pain.

Things can be just as frustrating at the doctor's office. We've seen that X-rays or other imaging tests often don't serve up a clear explanation of the pain. Many people assume that if there's not an anatomical explanation, it must look like an imaginary problem. I've heard the protest, "This isn't all in my head!" too many times.

Without a clear-cut diagnosis—even if it's wrong—you may feel that no one believes you, whether family, friends, or work associates. It may feel like they think you're malingering, imagining things, hypochondriacal, or exaggerating.

Sometimes people with back pain may feel pushed into aggressive therapy. The nudge may come from family members, bosses, or attorneys. Because it's an invisible pain, you may feel pressure to seek out imaging, opioids, injections, or even surgery as a means of demonstrating your commitment to getting better.

Furthermore, the pain can be so bad that it's hard to understand how a test could fail to pinpoint the cause. It may be hard to imagine that it could get better without surgery.

But remember the traps that JFK, General Fridovich, Cindy McCain, and Jerome Groopman fell into. Pursuing these interventions may not help, and they sometimes make things worse. One goal of treatment should be to avoid this quicksand.

So let's get something straight. It's not all in your head. The pain is in your back! Even if the X-rays don't show much, the pain is in your back. But the causes of the pain may be complex indeed.

We've seen that acute back pain tends to get better fast. Though we can't see this pain on imaging tests, it seems likely that much acute back pain is caused by problems in the ligaments and muscles that surround the vertebrae. There may be sprains or even tears in these structures. There may be muscle spasms. Muscle tension may increase as a mechanism to "guard" small, invisible injuries to discs or facets. In some ways, the pain is protecting *too well*—even when there's little or no tissue injury.

Like a sprained ankle, these problems can be extremely painful. Remember that Isaiah Thomas couldn't get out of bed one day—although he was playing NBA basketball the next. Sometimes it feels like something's broken. But these acute episodes tend to heal in a matter of days or a few weeks.

We also saw that even herniated discs tend to heal in a matter of months. They usually shrink on MRI scans over that time. If they contact a spinal nerve, they can cause nerve inflammation that results in pain. But that pain subsides as the inflammation, swelling, and heat subside.

If these tissues tend to heal, how do we explain pain that goes on for years?

The New Neuroscience

Pain evolved as a warning system, to alert us to the risk of tissue damage. There's a rare genetic disease in which the affected people experience no pain. That may sound like heaven, but the truth is far from it. These people sustain burns, fractures, lacerations, eye injuries, and destruction of their joints that the rest of us avoid precisely because we get the warnings of pain. Such people have a reduced life expectancy.

In our old way of thinking, pain was a purely physical phenomenon and always protective. Tissue injury stimulated a nerve that sent impulses to the spinal cord, then to a spot in the brain, and we perceived pain. This was the concept of René Descartes, the French philosopher and mathematician. It was insightful for the 1600s, but the concept is now four hundred years out of date.

A corollary of this centuries-old model was that when tissue healed, the pain stopped. So if you continue to have back pain, it would mean there's still tissue damage going on. That in turn might mean you shouldn't move too much and shouldn't exercise your back. It would need rest to heal.

This thinking led to recommending bed rest, time off work, and no lifting. We warned people not to run, not to play golf, not to lift more than twenty pounds. We had people walking on eggshells.

Even a recent study reflected this problem. One patient, describing instructions from a physical therapist, said, "She's told me more what nots to do than what to do." Another described his doctor's advice: "basically . . . that I shouldn't do any bending or lifting."

We often warned patients about the bulging disc, the degenerating facet joints, or the pinched nerve that showed up on imaging tests, presuming we had discovered the tissue damage causing the pain. But that was before we realized that those changes were so common in normal, pain-free people. Yet even now, people who know about these things on their MRI scans may hold back from certain activities for fear of making things worse.

An important feature of the old way of thinking was that the brain and spinal cord were unchanging in adults. Once you stopped growing, these organs had all the cells they were going to get. These cells didn't divide or change much. Additionally, in the old model, the brain only perceived pain, and never changed it.

Newer research on the spinal cord and brain has turned that thinking on its head.

The brain and the spinal cord turn out to be constantly changing. They do make new cells. The cells constantly rearrange their connections with other cells. Inside the cells, genes that were turned off get turned on and vice versa. That means new proteins get made and cell behavior can change. Scientists coined the term "neuroplasticity" to describe this ability of the brain and spinal cord to change.

An implication of this is that pain impulses from a painful back aren't just transmitted through a nerve to the spinal cord to be perceived at one place in the brain. Not only does the brain perceive pain, it can modify, or "modulate," pain.

Pain impulses can get amplified or tamped down along the way by other parts of the nervous system. If you're tired, frustrated, or stressed, impulses may get amplified as they travel through the spinal cord and inside the brain. If you're having a relaxing, wonderful time with the love of your life, the impulses may get tamped down. In other words, thoughts and feelings can have an important effect on pain. This process is termed "neural modulation."

Furthermore, when nerve impulses arrive in the brain, they don't stimulate just one spot. Instead, they tickle a complex network that involves many parts of the brain. Memories, anticipations, and moods get linked up with the pain, again in ways we're totally unaware of. The conscious mind is oblivious.

So the experience of pain is complex and variable. The same stimulus won't be experienced the same way every time, or the same way by different people. The spinal cord and the brain can increase or decrease sensitivity to pain in a process that we're completely unaware of. The spinal cord can act like the volume control on your sound system, with a knob that increases or decreases the loudness. But it does so without your knowing about it or controlling it.

Sometimes that complex network in the brain stays active even if there aren't pain impulses coming from the spine itself. One result is that sometimes pain isn't related to tissue injury, and sometimes it continues well beyond tissue healing. Sometimes the changes in the spinal cord and brain make pain sensations continue even if there aren't nerve signals coming from the back itself.

You feel the pain in the back, all right, but it may not be because of any tissue damage there. Scientists refer to this as "central sensitization" because it results from changes to the central nervous system—the brain and spinal cord—rather than to nerves in the spine itself.

Very recent research, using highly specialized brain imaging, suggests that there may also be structural features of the brain that predispose some people to develop ongoing pain. Though the results aren't yet definitive, it looks like these features may exist before the onset of pain.

These new observations help explain why some people develop persistent back pain without an explanation on the spinal MRI. Unfortunately, we can't see any of these changes in the spinal cord and the brain with routine MRI scans or X-rays.

Those tests aren't going to explain the pain, although newer functional MRI and PET scanning—still used mostly for research—may yet offer some insights. In fact, functional MRI is already revealing how brain activity due to pain can be modified by distraction, for example.

The problem in this situation isn't tissue damage. In this circumstance, the pain isn't protective. Indeed, it has no value.

But it's also not imaginary, or hypochondriacal, or due to mental weakness. In fact, susceptibility to this problem may be at least partly genetic.

Recent studies, for example, suggest that persistent neck pain after traffic accidents is associated with specific gene variants. These genes affect stress hormones, which in turn affect nerve cells and promote inflammation. Though the exact mechanisms are complex and still poorly understood, the problem is one of central sensitization and neural modulation, not hypochondriasis. Similarly, the structural features of the brain we noted above seem to exist before the onset of pain, and we have no control over them.

Here it's worth remembering a lesson from General Fridovich. Prescription opioids may help to reduce the pain in acute pain situations, such as after an operation. But in the long term, they may actually increase the problem of central sensitization. As a result, opioids are rarely a major part of the solution, but they're often a major part of the problem.

The Evolution and Resolution of Persistent Pain

Here's a scenario that may be familiar to some people with persistent pain. It's a sequence of events that's been described by pain experts who treat military veterans.

When you first go to a doctor or other health care professional for back pain, you're in a hopeful phase. You're expecting to get better, and you try some straightforward treatments. Maybe it's pain medications, maybe it's physical therapy, and maybe it involves referral to some specialists.

But if there's not much improvement, you may enter a doubtful phase. You suspect that your doctor and your family are wondering if you have "real pain." You may start demanding more. Tests get repeated. You seek more and more aggressive treatments.

Maybe that means more opioids or injections. Maybe back surgery. Maybe repeat back surgery. MRI findings may drive your doctor to recommend treatments that are destined to offer little benefit. In this phase, you make decisions out of frustration. Sometimes you may pursue treatments just to validate the problem, to prove to people around you that it's "real." And some of these may just lead to more problems. It's hard to think things through in a careful, deliberate way.

If things still aren't working out well, you may enter a hopeless phase. You're convinced that your doctors are the problem. They're convinced that you're the problem. There's a process of rejection going on, and perhaps the whole process starts again, with a new set of doctors.

What do experts recommend to avoid this vicious cycle? How can we restore hope?

One step is to veer from searching for The Cause of the pain to identifying its effects. In part, this means accepting ambiguous results from tests. We've seen that MRI scans and similar tests often fail to provide clear answers for a cause and can even generate red herrings. Getting yet more tests, or repeating the ones you've had, is unlikely to help.

Focusing on effects rather than causes means examining the ways you may have limited your activities or withdrawn from normal roles. Examining fears that may have evolved and things that you now avoid. It means concentrating on living as full a life as possible. As a doctor-blogger writes, "The choice may be ruling over the disease or being ruled by it."

This refocus goes along with a shift in treatment goals. Rather than concentrate on curing the symptom of pain, the emphasis settles on restoring daily function and improving quality of life. This may sound like a dodge, but most people find that this refocus ends up reducing pain as well. It's a mistake to believe that the pain has to be relieved first.

The shift in treatment goals has another important implication. You can't stand by passively while you wait for a doctor or other health professional to bestow The Cure upon you. There are no silver bullets here. Getting better requires assuming a more active role and more responsibility for making treatment decisions. We'll discuss ways of doing that later on.

All these steps acknowledge that back pain isn't a straightforward disease with a definitive cure, like appendicitis. Instead, it's a complex problem that can become an ongoing challenge, just like diabetes or high blood pressure. Like other chronic conditions, it can require lifestyle changes, family engagement, workplace changes, and continuing effort.

For those of us in the health care professions, it requires a mental shift as well. Rather than pose as experts with The Answer, we need to shift our role toward that of teacher and coach. Rather than pretend that a pill, procedure, or program is going to solve the problem, we have to acknowledge that the keys usually lie in what patients can do for themselves.

That often means helping to facilitate self-management in a collaborative effort. And we need to accept that for some patients, we'll have to continue that effort over a long time, just as we do with diabetes or high blood pressure.

This isn't the same as saying "just live with it" or "get used to it." It's saying there's often no quick fix, and improvement may require a sustained effort.

Got Stress?

Got any stress in your life these days? Long commutes alongside kamikaze drivers in wretched traffic? Kids that talk back? Problems at work? Job insecurity? Deadlines? Financial worries? A leak in the roof? Relationship problems? Is there anybody who doesn't have stress in his or her life these days? Now add back pain, and it's a particularly toxic brew.

How do you respond to stress? If you're like lots of people, you sometimes get headaches when things are most stressful. I do. Sometimes, though, it's aching in my left shoulder from tense muscles. Actually, it's more like my upper back. For some people, it's the lower back. For some people, it's the digestive system. Most of us seem to have a target organ where stress expresses itself.

Stress probably didn't cause your back pain in the first place, but it probably makes the pain worse. It's one of those things that affects your spinal cord and brain in a way that turns up the amplifier. The amplified pain can make you fearful of certain activities and lead you to avoid them.

This is part of the rationale behind a treatment called cognitive-behavioral therapy. This is something your doctor may recommend, and your immediate response may be, "I don't need a shrink. I'm not crazy."

Indeed, you're not crazy. Fear and avoidance of activities aren't signs of mental illness or weakness. They're normal responses to painful experiences. There's no diagnosis of fear or avoidance in the *Diagnostic and Statistical Manual*, which is the bible of psychiatric diagnosis. But fear and avoidance can ruin your life.

Cognitive-behavioral therapy isn't traditional psychotherapy. It's more of an effort to reeducate, retrain, and reframe your thinking and behavior regarding back pain. Your primary care doctor, your chiropractor, or your physical therapist may all contribute to the process, even if they don't call it that. Some health care systems are experimenting with telephone versions or even online forms of it. Don't expect to lie on the proverbial psychiatrist's couch or to have a long and drawn-out course.

Nonetheless, cognitive-behavioral therapy may sometimes involve referral to a psychologist, psychiatrist, or other mental health professional. As long as that's someone trained in pain management, don't recoil. Because it often helps. And as we'll see, it can be a valuable adjunct to exercise and other therapy.

The overall goal of cognitive-behavioral therapy is to help you reverse the negative impacts of pain on your life and to gain control over the pain. It aims to help change behaviors that increase stress and tension, reduce physical activity, and aggravate pain.

Typical components are training about pacing your activities and dealing with problems related to sleep, fatigue, and irritability. Cognitive-behavioral therapy provides self-management strategies for controlling pain, including relaxation techniques that help to deal with stress. It also helps you learn ways to reduce depression and anxiety caused by the pain.

An important aim is increasing participation in social, recreational, home, and work activities that are important to you. The focus is on identifying your most important goals and working together to reduce barriers to those goals.

In some settings, this educational and problem-solving strategy is paired with strategies for increasing movement and physical activity, often with supervision from a physical therapist. We'll talk more about exercise in a later chapter.

This may all sound a little soft and a little "New Age" to some people. Or still too much like "it's all in your head." Or like it's giving up on a cure.

But see here: dozens of randomized trials have shown benefits in treating persistent pain. The strategies you can learn often aren't intuitively obvious. In some research studies, the combination of cognitive-behavioral therapy and exercise therapy was as effective as spinal fusion surgery for treating people with worn-out discs.

In fact, it appears that this combination of cognitive-behavioral therapy and exercise can literally change your brain. It appears to "reprogram" the pain circuitry, perhaps like rebooting your computer when it acts up. Only this is a slower process, and requires more work. This is something drugs and surgery can't do. The result is less pain, more activity, and better quality of life.

Part of the goal is to give control over symptoms back to you rather than your doctors. Too often, people begin to feel powerless in the face of persistent pain, and feel they depend entirely on prescriptions, injections, or procedures that someone else must provide. This can reinforce feelings of helplessness.

The combination of cognitive-behavioral therapy and exercise puts you firmly in control. These are skills that are available to you after office hours and on weekends. They don't require monthly refills. Now what does the exercise part of this combination look like?

Chapter 13

BOOT CAMP

Attorney Eric Stevens (not his real name) loved running and had competed in six marathons. He also loved playing with his five kids, skiing, fly-fishing, and ocean surfing. But the summer after he turned forty-five, he moved some furniture and he was also sneezing a lot with allergies. He's not sure what the real culprit was, but one night he began to have excruciating back pain that traveled into his left buttock and leg.

He couldn't stay in bed so he slithered to the floor, and then couldn't get off the floor. Somehow he got to the emergency room, got some pain medication, and gradually improved over a few days. But he had lingering numbness in his left foot that bothered him when he ran.

After referral to an orthopedic surgeon he respected, Stevens had an MRI of his back. As we might expect, it showed several abnormalities, including a narrowed disc, a bulging disc, and moderate narrowing of the spinal canal called spinal stenosis. Also, a protruding disc appeared to be impinging on a spinal nerve. In addition, Stevens's ankle reflex on the left side was gone.

Stevens reported that the orthopedic surgeon told him he "absolutely, positively" needed a decompression operation and a spine fusion but could start running three months after surgery.

Stevens sought a second opinion from a neurosurgeon, who recommended *against* surgery but told Stevens to stop running altogether. He said that if Stevens did have a fusion operation, he would have to stop running for one to two years because it takes that long to heal. So much for professional consensus!

Stevens became the rare case who gets written up in a medical journal and discussed by national experts. Dr. James Weinstein, an orthopedic surgeon from Dartmouth Medical School, was able to offer a third opinion. He discouraged surgery and said, "I would not dissuade Mr. S from running. . . . In fact, unless his symptom pattern changes, I would encourage it."

In a follow-up article a year later, Stevens commented, "I am doing great. I decided not to have surgery and my back has been fine. I still have the numbness in my left foot and calf, but it doesn't really bother me. I am running 25 to 34 miles a week in preparation to run the Boston Marathon in April. I have never felt better."

Confronted with back pain, many people are afraid to exercise. Especially if there are worrisome things on an MRI scan, many people imagine that exercise can only make it worse. Stevens's greatest concern was whether it was safe to resume running and what would happen if he didn't have surgery.

In the face of pain and MRI abnormalities, it seems counterintuitive that vigorous exercise could be safe, much less good for you. Yet Eric Stevens found that resuming exercise made him feel better and worry less.

Stevens was physically active and dedicated to exercise before he got back pain. And after the initial episode, his main symptom was numbness more than pain. So perhaps he was naturally inclined and favorably disposed toward resuming a rigorous exercise regimen. Furthermore, he'd experienced acute rather than persistent pain, another factor in his favor.

Most people aren't marathoners, and most of us are more sedentary at our best than Eric Stevens was at his worst. And many people find that back pain restricts their activities even further.

Remember our earlier discussion about Dr. Jerome Groopman, and recall that we left him after two unsuccessful back operations and nineteen years of severe activity limitation. His was truly a case of persistent back pain. Here's how he described his situation:

> Like most patients who have undergone spinal fusions, I continued to have persistent lower-back pain afterward: I couldn't run, I couldn't drive for long stretches, I couldn't carry heavy grocery bags.
>
> When my sons were in grade school, I wanted to teach them to play baseball, but swinging a bat triggered sharp pain in my back, and I retreated to the sidelines. . . . There were periods of respite . . . but then an apparently innocuous movement would cause my lumbar area to explode in spasm. I never knew when or where it might happen. Along with unpredictable pain came its companion, a sense of prevailing fear.

Frustrated and with worsening pain, Groopman sought the advice of a rheumatologist, a specialist in joint and arthritis problems. The rheumatologist in turn referred Groopman to a rehabilitation doctor in Boston, Dr. Jim Rainville.

Rainville practices at the New England Baptist Hospital, the same hospital where John Kennedy had his first back operation. JFK's youngest brother, Senator Edward Kennedy, had received care there after a plane crash and a spinal fracture. Basketball legend Larry Bird had undergone surgery and rehabilitation there. But many of Rainville's patients weren't celebrities; they were ordinary people and elderly adults with back pain.

Rainville ran a rehabilitation program that had acquired a reputation as a boot camp. Groopman went to see him with trepidation and described the initial visit. After carefully reviewing Groopman's medical history, examination, and MRI, Rainville declared that he was "worshiping the volcano god of pain . . . the god of pain is your master." He went on to say, "I believe you can be freed from your pain. I believe you can rebuild yourself and do much, much more."

Groopman recalled to me that Rainville walked him to the "gym," where physical therapists were working with people who had persistent back pain. He described seeing a seventy-five-year-old grandmother carrying a crate of metal bricks. And Rainville telling him, "Two months ago she couldn't walk because of back pain."

This alone was motivating to Groopman and was a part of what Rainville calls "modeling." The idea is that positive actions of one patient help shape the attitudes and expectations of other patients.

Finally, Rainville threw down a challenge. "It's your choice: to try or not to try. You can walk out of my office now and believe everything you've believed for the past nineteen years, and live the way you have. Or you can test me. And I'll tell you now, I'm right." Groopman described Rainville's introduction as "shock and awe."

Dr. Groopman couldn't imagine that a rigorous rehabilitation program would help, and he thought it would surely make his pain worse. He told me that he had undergone physical therapy years earlier, after his spine surgery. At that time, the physical therapists told him that if something caused pain, he should stop.

Yet Rainville had offered a glimmer of hope that was refreshing and that ultimately hooked Groopman, who decided to enroll in the program.

The physical therapists started him with three weeks of stretching exercises at home, a prelude to more vigorous exercise. He was so debilitated at that point that Groopman found even the stretching to be exhausting.

And when he actually began the supervised training, Groopman wrote, "Each exercise caused shooting pains in my back that ran down my buttocks, thighs, and feet. The therapists were unmoved by my pains, telling me firmly to keep challenging my body. I would leave the sessions depleted, needing to rest for hours, lying in bed on ice packs." He told me, "Rainville was like Simon Legree."

Despite plenty of skepticism, Groopman stayed focused on hopes for returning to his favorite activities. And an amazing thing began to happen over the next three months: "the constant pain became intermittent, then rare." He began to walk progressively longer distances, then to hike in the hills. Each increase in activity was accompanied by "days of spasm and pain, but I tried to ignore it all."

After a year, Groopman found that the daily pains were essentially gone. "I felt reborn. It seemed almost magical," he wrote. He still has occasional back pain, and says he still has some limits, but he is able to be far more active.

And he still exercises. He described his regimen to me: swimming three days a week, walking every morning for one and a half to two miles, and bicycling three times a week.

In retrospect, he describes the hardest part of this transformation as taking the very first step. "Fear is often the most significant hurdle—fear of pointless pain and suffering." He noted that even small changes early in the process gave him some hope, and he believes that in itself was a major part of recovery. He found that hope helped to improve pain, which in turn increased hope and created a virtuous cycle of improvement.

What Happened Here?

Jim Rainville is of medium height with a solid, muscular build. He has some thinning hair at the temples, where it's also graying. He practiced family medicine on the faculty at Brown University while also in private practice for six years. He describes back pain as the biggest problem in that practice. Perhaps driven by that experience, he returned to medical training, but this time in rehabilitation medicine. Now his practice is largely with people who have back pain, like Jerome Groopman.

When he talks about his work, Rainville is intense and animated. He's a friend, and we've recently been working together on a task force dealing with research standards for back pain, sponsored by the National Institutes of Health. This gave me a chance to quiz him one evening about his approach.

Rainville believes that the degenerative changes we see on MRI scans in the spinal discs and facet joints are important, but that there's a highly idiosyncratic relationship between these changes and pain perception. Meaning that some people are significantly bothered with pain while others aren't.

He argues that people with persistent back pain have a "lowered stimulus threshold," meaning that a given stimulus provokes a response from neurons in the spinal cord and brain earlier than expected. Like the neuroscientists, he notes that persistent low back pain isn't protective and has no value.

Rainville sees that many people begin to avoid exercise and activity due to pain, as Groopman described. He also finds that modern lifestyles aggravate the problem of back pain. That's because there's essentially no *need* to exercise or use the back for vigorous activities.

He cautions that many people turn to opioid medications for pain relief, but he finds this an impediment to improving persistent pain. He says that patients using regular opioids don't improve in his program, with "almost no exceptions."

But he argues that we can change how neurons function if they're stimulated repeatedly and willingly. Exercise then becomes a way to change pain sensitivity. Rainville refers to this as a way of reeducating the nervous system.

This is consistent with some of the surprising concepts of the new neuroscience we discussed earlier. The brain and spinal cord can change. Groopman notes that this is a reversal of our usual "mind-body" concept, and more of a "body-mind" concept. That is, not only does the mind affect the body, but also what happens in the body has an important effect on the brain.

Rainville says a journalist was the first to use the name "boot camp" to describe his program, and the name stuck. Rainville likes it. He believes it's important that patients feel they've earned their improvement, and earned it with dignity. To this end, he believes the program has to be both physically and psychologically challenging.

Rainville is quick to acknowledge that anxiety and fear are important components of persistent pain, just as Groopman described in himself. But Rainville feels that mental health specialists sometimes make the mistake of simply asking patients to accept major limitations. He wants instead to change the mindset to "you can do it."

From the outset, Rainville's program ruffled feathers and challenged the conventional wisdom. As Groopman described in his earlier physical therapy program, the usual approach has been to say, "If it hurts, don't do it." A common saying was, "Let pain be your guide." Consistent with the newer concepts of neuroscience, Rainville turned that philosophy on its head. He argues that if a careful evaluation shows no major structural damage or underlying disease, it's important to push to certain physical goals, even in the face of pain. Rainville explains to patients that although pain may be debilitating, it's not a sign that they're doing themselves harm.

When the program started, members of the local physical therapy community criticized it. They argued that the program failed to provide precise physiological diagnoses and offered a "cookbook" approach. But over the years, Rainville's program came to be seen as a successful group and a desirable place to work.

Is There Science behind Exercise Therapy?

For people with acute back pain—new in the past few weeks—specific back exercises don't seem to help. However, neither does bed rest. The best advice in this situation is to continue walking and continue normal daily activities as much as possible. After the acute phase subsides, though, exercise is valuable to help prevent recurring episodes of back pain.

For persistent back pain—pain that's gone on for more than three months—the situation is different. Here back exercises seem to make a difference, and they become the mainstay of therapy. They even help people return to work faster.

There have been dozens of randomized trials comparing various exercise programs with routine care alone, back pain education, instruction in lifting techniques, or other treatment approaches. Though the average effect is modest, the results are consistent. Exercise seems to reduce pain and improve daily functioning more than those comparison treatments.

Here I'll speculate that the sort of boot camp approach Rainville advocates may be more effective than less demanding exercise efforts. Though we don't have proof, perhaps the more rigorous approach achieves better results than the modest effects in many studies.

After any initial exercise therapy, what style of exercise works best for long-term benefits? Here the studies fail to show much difference among competing exercise programs. For long-term use, Jim Rainville says, "Zumba, yoga, Pilates—I don't care." He feels all are helpful.

Research studies on stretching exercises, yoga, Pilates, the Alexander Technique, Tai Chi, water aerobics, and plain old aerobic exercise on dry ground all show benefits. None is clearly superior to the others.

So try any of them. Bicycle. Swim. Play your favorite sports. Books with exercise programs for back pain abound. The best advice is to choose the exercise approach you enjoy most and are most likely to stick with.

Why does exercise work? There are several theories, and all may have some validity. First, strengthening the muscles that surround the spine may improve support, provide more stamina for physical activities, and increase strength for everyday lifting. The experience of increasing activity alone may help reduce fear of movement. There also is good evidence that exercise helps ease depression, which often accompanies persistent pain.

As Rainville, Groopman, and neuroscientists argue, exercise may help "rewire" or "reeducate" the brain and the muscles. It may recalibrate the threshold for firing pain neurons in the spinal cord and brain. Further, exercise seems to reduce the frequency of repeat back pain, which is a common feature of the problem.

Finally, studies show that cognitive-behavioral therapy plus exercise works better than either one alone. Cognitive-behavioral therapy helps reduce the fear that pain with exercise means you're harming yourself.

It seems likely that this combination accelerates the "rewiring" process, and small improvements that result from either component reinforce the hope and the virtuous cycle that Groopman described. In retrospect, Groopman believes that the growing sense of hope he acquired was at least as important as improvement in actual fitness.

In fact, several studies suggest that the benefits of exercise may be only weakly related to measurable changes in muscle strength or endurance. This again argues for important changes that may be occurring in the nerves, spinal cord, and brain.

Of course, exercise seems to be on every doctor's and public health official's list of great ideas. It almost seems like a default recommendation, an addendum to every treatment plan. There are lots of reasons to exercise. It's good for your heart; it's good for your lungs; it's good for improving sleep; it's good for your intestinal tract. It slows down aging. It's good for keeping your weight down, and that may add to the benefits for back pain.

The challenge with exercise, of course, is getting motivated to do it. I know I love finding excuses not to go to the gym or to go running. Given a choice between settling in to watch Sunday afternoon football with pretzels and beer or going to the gym, I suspect many of us would find reasons to settle in with Rover in our laps. It's raining. It's cold out. I need to hold my own when my buddies talk about the game around the water cooler.

But relieving back pain happens faster than all those other health benefits of exercise. It might take twenty years for exercise to prevent a heart attack or slow the aging process. But with back pain, you often see the benefits in a matter of weeks, which may be more motivating. And besides, you can usually watch the game at the gym.

Some studies suggest that exercise works best when supervised, as it was for JFK and for Jerome Groopman. You might legitimately interrupt here and say, "Yeah, but they could afford it." The truth is that it's easier with most insurance plans to get an MRI or a spinal fusion operation than to get coverage for physical therapy. Gym memberships won't be covered at all. Indeed, this creates a policy agenda that we'll discuss later. But you may at least be able to get professional advice that will get you started.

Buying into the combination of rigorous exercise and cognitive-behavioral therapy may sound like eating your broccoli. Good for you, maybe, but no fun. And it doesn't make you feel instantly better. Most of us are more inclined to look for the quick fix, and we're attracted to high-tech solutions.

My colleague Donald Patrick and I coined the term "techno-consumption" in an earlier book. We argued that Americans are in love with their technological gadgets. This is most obvious with our computers, electronic notepads, smartphones, and Wi-Fi hotspots. It extends to home electronics like our sound systems, flat-screen TVs, digital video recorders, and digital cameras.

And it extends to medical technology as well. The allure of an artificial disc, the latest spinal screw implant, or an electronic spinal cord stimulator is almost irresistible. Or it might be a bone growth stimulator, a TENS unit, a new drug, or a new needling technique that attracts us.

Exercise and cognitive-behavioral therapy sound paltry, weak, and slow by comparison. But the high-tech solutions often prove disappointing and often pose significant risks. The low-tech interventions have stronger and more consistent evidence behind them.

What is Jerome Groopman's advice to people with persistent back pain? After his nineteen years of debilitating pain, then a sojourn in a challenging boot camp? He says to find a doctor you like—preferably a rehabilitation specialist who's part of the new school of neuroscience and exercise science. He acknowledges that not everyone wants a shock-and-awe, Simon Legree personality like the one Jim Rainville presented to him, though he feels he needed it. He says to evolve a regular exercise program and combine it with cognitive-behavioral therapy, delivered by any approach.

The point is that with these interventions, persistent back pain is treatable—even if we don't have the definitive cure. Recall that Kennedy, Fridovich, and Groopman all continued to experience some back pain, even after their successful treatments. But they enjoyed big improvements in quality of life and were no longer controlled by their pain.

These may be key steps toward taking control of the situation yourself. Are there other ways you can take control?

Chapter 14

AMPLIFYING YOUR VOICE

Some medical decisions are easy. Other than some people who are terminally ill, almost everyone would want antibiotics for pneumonia. Nearly everyone would want thyroid hormone treatment if he or she had symptomatic hypothyroidism. If you have iron deficiency anemia, taking oral iron tablets is cheap, easy, and effective. Who wouldn't want to set a broken bone?

But most treatments for low back pain are more complicated. They aren't lifesaving. In the absence of severe spine trauma, infection, cancer, or extremely rare circumstances, they aren't preventing paralysis. There's a wide variety of options for pain relief, and there's rarely one dominant approach. Many treatments have potential major complications. Furthermore, passively expecting a pill, procedure, or program to cure back pain is unrealistic. Instead, patients need to become actively involved in their own care and decisions about it.

This is an area of medicine where the decisions are rarely black and white; they're almost always gray. Consider surgery for a herniated disc that's causing both back pain and sciatica. Unless you're having incontinence of your bladder or bowels, weakness in both legs, or steadily worsening leg weakness in addition to pain, surgery isn't aimed at preventing neurologic damage. Instead, it's aimed at pain relief.

For carefully selected patients—those with symptoms, examination findings, and imaging results that all line up, and no response to several weeks of nonsurgical care—removal of a herniated disc can result in prompt pain relief.

But what if you don't have surgery? We noted earlier that herniated discs tend to shrink over time. And the pain tends to shrink over time as well. It takes longer than with surgery. But over some period—usually a year or two—most patients improve just as much even without surgery. What about numbness, or missing reflexes, or minor foot weakness? Those seem to recover at about the same pace with or without surgery.

And while disc surgery is successful most of the time, it's no guarantee. Remember the experience of Jerome Groopman with his first operation for a herniated disc. Poor outcomes may be a result of uncertainty about the cause of pain, even with modern imaging. They may result from scarring that develops after surgery. They may result from complications during surgery. One predictor of bad results is depression, even though that might seem unrelated to surgical problems. Sometimes the reason for bad results just isn't clear.

So should someone in this situation have surgery or not? There's no one right answer.

In one camp are people who would jump at the chance for surgery. These people are desperate for immediate relief, can't concentrate on anything else, and are happy to accept the uncertainties and risks of surgery. When carefully advised about the options, they'd choose surgery in a heartbeat.

Others, equally well informed, may see it in a completely different way. They may feel that with other pain control measures, they can put up with it while natural healing proceeds. They may be able to adjust work activities to avoid postures and situations that aggravate the pain. They may find the risks of surgery unacceptable, and the pain manageable. For people in this camp, later surgery is always an option if they don't get better. Delayed surgery appears to be generally as effective as earlier surgery.

People in both camps are right! This is a situation where reasonable, well-informed people might come to completely different decisions, based on their own values and preferences.

So, to get the right treatment, you have to be involved. But your involvement isn't meaningful if you aren't well informed about the options. Studies suggest that people who are most confident about their medical choices are often not well informed. How do you get well informed?

Making Informed Decisions

Although market rhetoric pervades discussions of health care, this isn't remotely a market like the one for buying a car or a digital TV. One reason is that you, the consumer, usually have little idea what you're buying when it comes to medical care.

You have some concept of the differences between a Mercedes-Benz and a Ford Fiesta. You know the trade-offs in cost, comfort, and amenities. That's because you've bought and driven cars before, seen these models on the street, and read reviews in the newspaper or consumer magazines. The prices are on the stickers. You may be able to quibble a bit, but you have a pretty good idea of what you're going to pay.

But when it comes to a spine operation, a medial branch neurotomy, or even long-term opioid therapy, who really knows what they're buying? Most people have no experience with these things, yet the stakes in the decision are high.

Try as you might, finding prices is near impossible. Recent disclosures make it clear that the price may vary fourfold for the same procedure in different facilities, though you'd have a hard time finding that out.

More often than not, you're dependent on expert advice regarding medical treatments. Unfortunately, as we've seen, doctors sometimes recommend pain treatments that aren't terribly effective or in circumstances when they're unlikely to help. Studies suggest that treatments are sometimes less effective or more risky than patients realize. Doctors frequently make treatment recommendations, often for pet therapies, without making the range of options clear. Doctors rarely have a good knowledge of your personal values and preferences. Sometimes doctors have conflicts of interest.

We've described some effective treatments in earlier chapters, so it's rarely the case that you have no choice of therapy. But when doctors fail to mention alternatives to their recommendations, patients aren't aware of their choices. Remember the title of our 1994 research study, "Who You See Is What You Get."

Informed Consent

What about the informed consent process? When a procedure is recommended to you, there's always a form to sign that explains its benefits and risks. Those forms often include a long list of dire things that can occasionally go wrong. Doesn't this ensure that you're well informed?

Unfortunately, those consent forms rarely discuss all the benefits and risks of the alternatives. They rarely describe what's likely to happen if you don't have the procedure. They don't usually say exactly what "common" or "rare" means. Is a rare complication one in ten or one in ten thousand?

Some researchers have studied what happens in doctors' offices when treatment decisions are being made. This is done, for example, with tape recordings of the conversations, with both the doctor's and the patient's consent. These studies find that even if doctors discuss the options, they less often discuss the risks and benefits and rarely check to see how well patients understand.

Indeed, "informed consent" often takes the form of persuading a patient to agree with a recommendation rather than providing a balanced discussion of the options.

Other Sources of Patient Information

What about information you find on the web, where it seems you can find answers to everything? Sadly, the quality of medical information on the Internet varies all over the map. Much of the information is intended to sell a particular product, approach, hospital, or medical group. The medical experts whose comments appear on many websites have their own pet treatments, and benefit from them. Many have conflicts of interest over certain products, as we've seen in the case of kickbacks for using certain drugs or devices. As we noted earlier, the drug and device companies are unlikely to provide balanced or complete information.

How about the patient education brochures and handouts in your doctor's office? Patients typically describe these materials as being either too simple or too technical. They often find that the materials don't address treatments they're interested in. And these materials often have too little information on treatment effectiveness, alternative treatments, uncertainties, and self-care. Specialists report that the materials often give a false impression of treatment efficacy, tending to exaggerate benefits and minimize risks.

And the news media? Reports on back pain have an ugly habit of describing "breakthroughs." Unfortunately, I've seen breakthroughs on back pain reported in the press every few months for the past twenty-five years. And over those twenty-five years, rates of disability from back pain have only gotten worse. Journalists themselves acknowledge sometimes overstating medical findings in order to get more attention for a story.

And medical researchers often abet this process by exaggerating the importance of their own work. Researchers like a little taste of celebrity like everyone else. One medical researcher told a news reporter that getting his name on the front page of the *New York Times* was the only recognition that came close to winning a Nobel Prize. Furthermore, media attention may help researchers get more funding and may help the agencies that provide the funding. It's also good for the researchers' hospitals, universities, or research institutes.

Where *can* you turn for accurate and useful information?

Decision Aids

There's growing interest among doctors and hospitals in facilitating a process of shared decision making between doctors and patients. This doesn't mean making medical decisions on your own, but it also doesn't mean passively accepting every doctor's advice. Instead, it truly means *shared* decision making.

For this to be meaningful, you need to know when there's more than one choice. And that there's a legitimate choice: reasonable people might choose differently. The doctor should know the medical facts better than you do, but only you know your personal values and preferences.

And for any medical treatment or procedure, you ought to know these things before making a decision:

- What *are* your other options?
- What are the likely benefits of each, and how big are those benefits?
- What are the most common and the most serious risks of each option?
- What will happen if you don't have the treatment?

One strategy for providing such information is the use of so-called decision aids. Yes, these are patient education materials. But rather than blandly describe a treatment or imply a preferred course, they focus on the actual decision. These are most helpful in the gray areas of medicine, where there's no one right answer—exactly the situation with most back treatments.

These decision aids can take many forms: written materials, audio recordings, video presentations, or web-based presentations. Some are interactive so you can provide your age, diagnosis, and severity of the problem and receive tailored information. Some include exercises to help clarify your own values about the benefits and harms.

These programs, done right, make use of the best available research evidence for each treatment option. This strategy avoids introducing the biases of advocates for one treatment approach or another.

Finding these decision aids was still a challenge in 2013. If you're lucky, your health plan may contract with an organization that provides materials like this. It's worth asking both your insurance carrier and your doctor's office, and taking advantage of the materials if they're available.

Several organizations produce and distribute high-quality decision aids. Many are nonprofit organizations like the Informed Medical Decisions Foundation in Boston or Healthwise, based in Boise, Idaho. By way of *my* full disclosure, I need to say that I have been on the Board of Directors of the Informed Medical Decisions Foundation, and I confess that I'm partial to their materials.

What's the effect of these formal decision aids? There's now a solid research base from randomized trials to gauge their effects. By 2012, there were some 115 randomized trials of decision aids for a wide variety of medical conditions.

Combined, these studies show that decision aids improve patient knowledge of their options and result in more realistic treatment expectations. They help people reach choices more consistent with their informed values and prompt greater participation in decision making. And they seem to improve doctor-patient communication rather than detract from it. Overall, for elective surgery, decision aids tend to reduce the choice for surgery in favor of other options.

Decision Aids for Back Surgery

With regard to treatments for back pain, I'm aware of decision aids only for back surgery. We can hope that decision aids for various types of injections and drug therapy will follow.

What effects do the back surgery decision aids have? Several years ago, I worked with colleagues at the University of Washington, Group Health in Seattle, the University of Iowa, and the Informed Medical Decisions Foundation to produce and test decision aids targeting three conditions:

1. Herniated discs causing back pain and sciatica
2. Spinal stenosis, a condition in which the spinal canal becomes narrowed and pinches nerves
3. Back pain alone, often attributed to worn-out discs

These programs were computer-based and included a cartoon depiction of the spinal conditions being described. They also had video interviews with real patients who'd had good outcomes of surgery and people who'd had less favorable outcomes. There also were interviews with patients who experienced either good or bad outcomes from nonsurgical care. This provided the viewer with a vicarious sense of a range of possible results.

The programs included a tabulation of benefits and risks of both surgical and nonsurgical choices, based on the scientific literature as well as insurance claims databases.

The information was tailored to an individual's specific age and diagnosis. The programs included core segments for everyone to watch and optional segments that provided more information to those who wanted it. The optional segments covered topics such as spine imaging tests, chiropractic treatments, and drug therapy.

Initial testing of the program showed that patients at five medical facilities rated the program easy to understand and interesting to watch. Most liked the amount of information and thought the discussion of surgical versus nonsurgical treatment was completely balanced. Fewer patients remained undecided about treatment after watching the program than before.

We then undertook a randomized trial, comparing the computer-based video program with a written booklet that had similar information but no patient interviews or interactive features. We did the study in two locations: a neurosurgery practice at Group Health Cooperative in Seattle and an orthopedic spine clinic at the University of Iowa. Surgeons in both places were already relatively cautious about recommending surgery.

We found that patients had greater knowledge gains with the video program than with the booklet, especially among those with low initial knowledge about spine surgery. Patients gave higher scores to the video program regarding understandability, amount of information, and help in making decisions.

When it came to the actual choice of surgical or nonsurgical treatment, there were some interesting nuances. Among patients with a herniated disc, those who saw the video program chose less surgery: 32 percent compared with 47 percent of those who had only the booklet. We speculated that the favorable information about recovery without surgery led to a choice of less surgery.

However, among patients with spinal stenosis, those who saw the video program were more likely to choose surgery: 39 percent versus 29 percent of those with just the written materials. Here we speculated that the choice of more surgery was related to information that improvement was less likely with nonsurgical care.

Among those with back pain alone, those who saw the video program were substantially less likely to choose surgery, but the numbers were too small for us to draw firm conclusions. Overall, patients who saw the video program were less likely to choose surgery than those who just had the booklet.

But the most important results had to do with pain relief, improved activity levels, and return to work a year later. Here the results were virtually the same between groups, even though the video group received less surgery overall. In fact, pain relief was a bit better in the video group. Thus, it seems that choosing less surgery in the video group did no harm in terms of end results.

Overall, our conclusion was that patients who saw the video decision aid were better informed and chose less surgery but had equally good recovery. We also concluded that the video program influenced the choice of surgery in specific ways, depending on the patient's diagnosis.

The information in these decision aids has changed over time, as the producers incorporate new research findings. And there are good decision aids for back surgery besides the ones we pioneered.

So far, decision aids like this have not been widely available, but that's changing along with other aspects of health reform. Furthermore, there aren't yet good decision aids for many of the nonsurgical choices you may face. There are some formidable barriers to wider use, which we'll examine in the next chapter.

But growing demand from consumers would be a valuable spur to the development of more high-quality decision aids and their incorporation as a routine part of clinical practice. "Nothing about me without me" has become a rallying cry for those seeking greater patient involvement in their own health care decisions.

Perhaps someday we can move away from the passive concept of "informed consent," in which a patient simply consents to the doctor's recommendation. We could move instead toward the active concept of "informed request," in which well-informed patients request their treatment of choice. What changes do we need in our health and insurance systems to promote the sort of active involvement in care that this book advocates?

Chapter 15

SOME POLICY IMPLICATIONS

Current trends in the treatment of back pain suggest that we doctors aren't following clinical guidelines that are based on the best available science. In fact, clinical practice seems to be diverging further and further from evidence-based recommendations. This is especially remarkable for imaging, opioid prescribing, injections, and spinal fusion surgery.

The problem of limited guideline adherence is pervasive in medicine, and not just in the back pain world. There are many reasons why doctors might not follow a set of guidelines.

Doctors are overwhelmed with new information these days. It takes a lot of time to stay informed, and they may simply be unaware of recent guidelines. Beyond that, they may be skeptical about a guideline, disagree with it, mistrust the guideline developer, or simply feel it doesn't apply to a particular patient.

Doctors may fear that following a particular guideline will frustrate patients, especially if it suggests minimal testing or non-invasive treatment. Doctors worry that this will increase their risk of a malpractice lawsuit. We often simply have long-standing habits or routines that are hard to change.

Sometimes doctors face conflicting guidelines, as we saw in the case of spinal injections. But you may also recall publicity over conflicting guidelines in other areas of medicine as well—such as breast cancer screening. In that situation, expert panels disagreed over the age at which women should begin to have routine mammograms and how often they should have them.

These conflicting guidelines often appear to result from guideline authors with conflicts of interest. That is, many guidelines are written by specialists who make their livings from a particular procedure or who have ties to drug or device manufacturers. It's no surprise that they tend to favor more services and more intensive use of drugs and devices.

The Institute of Medicine has established new standards for writing guidelines, intended to minimize some of these conflicts. They emphasize the importance of having guideline panels that represent multiple medical and scientific specialties. They call for a panel chair with no conflicts of interest. They further indicate that most of the other panel members should not have conflicts of interest and that they should include a mix of clinicians, scientific experts, and lay members.

Sometimes we doctors face patient requests that conflict with the best scientific guidelines. This often takes the form of requesting more testing or more aggressive therapy than guidelines recommend. Again, many patients imagine that more health care can only be better.

In this situation, a doctor who follows the guidelines may risk an unhappy patient. Hospitals and health plans then create a dilemma for the doctor when they ask those patients to complete satisfaction questionnaires.

The doctor following the guidelines may get worse satisfaction scores. And in some health systems, this translates to less income for the doctor. This can create a financial incentive for providing unnecessary care.

In treating back pain, doctors report that ordering an MRI or prescribing an opioid is often the fastest way to stay on schedule and keep high satisfaction scores. We saw that patients who got a spinal imaging test were happier with their care than those who didn't—but also reported worse results.

Similarly, patients who are convinced they need opioids for pain may be dissatisfied if their doctors disagree. Unhappy patients respond not only with low satisfaction scores but also with bad ratings on doctor-grading websites. Explaining why an MRI or an opioid prescription may be unnecessary takes more time and risks unhappy patients. So doctors sometimes meet patient requests even if they seem ill-advised.

Given this array of problems, some solutions need to be aimed at the individual doctor. To begin with, doctors and the public deserve the highest-quality guidelines—based on the best scientific evidence and free of conflicts of interest.

The growing use of electronic medical record systems may make it easier for doctors to stay up-to-date. That's because guideline recommendations can be embedded to appear just when they're needed. For example, they can alert doctors when a particular imaging test is unnecessary. New data systems that track prescriptions also make it easier to let doctors know when an opioid prescription may be dangerous—because of similar prescriptions from other doctors, excessive doses, or risky drug combinations.

Increasingly, doctors are employed by hospitals or large health care systems and must answer to their employers. The administrators of these programs should understand that greater patient satisfaction with care isn't necessarily the same as better health. They may need to adjust doctors' performance evaluations to relate to actual health outcomes rather than patient satisfaction alone. In the case of back pain, the health outcomes could include patient reports of ability to perform daily activities. Such an approach may help reduce unnecessary or ineffective care and avoidable costs.

Treating people with back pain requires a doctor's time. Assessing the symptoms, examining the patient, explaining the problem, discussing treatment options, and motivating behavior change require more than ten minutes.

Yet ten- or fifteen-minute visits are the norm in primary care because reimbursement for these activities is so meager. This means that doctors are often required to schedule as many appointments as humanly possible in the course of a workday.

This approach reflects the recent evolution of medical care from a service to a business. The same evolution has renamed patients "consumers" or "clients," emphasizing their purchasing power rather than their health needs. It's language that emphasizes the opportunity to sell something more than the need to heal. It's an evolution that doesn't serve patients well.

Our system has created an approach that has to change if we're going to improve the quality of care. Patients with persistent back pain deserve and require more time.

Beyond these challenges for the individual doctor and patient, we've seen some elements of our society and health care system that may work against good guidelines and good results. These include wishful thinking, profit-driven marketing, and perverse financial incentives. We might add a few things to that list: media hype, limited FDA regulations, and limited knowledge of scientific evidence on the part of both doctors and patients. Are there things we could do to address these factors and to make the health care system itself more effective and efficient in managing back pain?

Insurance Coverage

In almost every U.S. insurance plan, it's easier to get reimbursed for having an MRI or a spinal injection than it is for getting physical therapy. The same is true for supervised exercise or cognitive-behavioral therapy. Recall that this is the approach that reduces fear and avoidance, enhances pacing of activities, reduces fatigue, and encourages relaxation techniques.

Yet exercise and cognitive-behavioral therapy are the things that appear most helpful for managing persistent back pain. And they seem to be underused. Given existing financial incentives, these patterns of care should be no surprise.

Insurance coverage often drives what doctors recommend and what patients do. If imaging and surgery are covered, but exercise therapy isn't, we should expect to get more imaging and surgery and less exercise therapy.

On the receiving side, we doctors get reimbursed for our time much more handsomely when we're injecting or operating than when we're examining patients in the office, providing information, or discussing options.

Doctors aren't simply greedy. I don't think most are motivated primarily by money. But they're all economically rational. They will gravitate to activities that provide greater rewards, and reimbursement is one of those. Furthermore, their employers—the administrators of hospitals and health plans—consistently urge doctors to generate more income.

So if you want doctors to spend more time providing a careful examination, giving information, or discussing options, you might let them know that you value those activities. If you're unhappy with ten-minute visits for complex problems, would you advocate better reimbursement of your doctor's time for doing those things? This would create more time for those activities.

Similarly, insurance coverage for physical therapy and for talk—like cognitive-behavioral therapy—is often meager in comparison to other services. Better coverage of these options would make them more attractive and accessible to many patients.

On the flip side, we might consider reducing payment for certain invasive procedures. This would be most appropriate when any benefit is unclear. For example, some insurance plans have begun to limit coverage for spinal fusion operations in situations where they're unlikely to help. North Carolina Blue Cross recently imposed such limits on spine fusion surgery for degenerative discs, and some other insurance plans have followed suit.

Do such restrictions help or harm patients? Dr. Brook Martin is a health services researcher at Dartmouth and formerly a colleague of mine at the University of Washington. He designed and led us in a clever study of this question. We were able to compare surgery for workers' compensation patients in two states with contrasting coverage policies for spinal fusion surgery. We might call it a natural experiment.

Washington State's workers' comp system implemented restrictions on coverage for spine fusions to situations where the benefit was the clearest. It required more justification of reasons for performing fusion operations. It also put limits on how extensive the surgery could be, regarding number of vertebrae involved and invasiveness of the operation itself. Furthermore, the state imposed stricter criteria for performing a second or third back operation.

In contrast, California imposed fewer restrictions and provided more generous reimbursement for surgically implanted devices.

When we compared patients having fusion operations in the two states, we found that patients in California had higher rates of fusion surgery, higher complication rates, higher rates of repeat surgery, and higher costs. They were more likely to be readmitted to the hospital after surgery. Together these findings suggested that Washington's greater restrictions were leading to better results at a lower cost.

Another set of insurance needs relates to the use of opioid painkillers. Many patients who use these drugs for a long time become physically dependent on them, and others become frankly addicted. Many become deeply ambivalent about the drugs and their doctors. They're grateful for every refill of medication that staves off symptoms of withdrawal, but they resent the control that the medication has over their lives. Some complain that doctors never properly advised them about the risks. Some want to stop the drugs and seek help in stopping.

Some who use prescription opioids even turn to the street to buy pills or heroin. At a needle-exchange program for heroin addicts, 39 percent described getting "hooked" first on prescription-type opioids. The National Survey on Drug Use and Health suggested even a grimmer situation. In that survey, 79 percent of people who reported starting heroin use in the past year had previously abused prescription pain medication.

In part, this is because of the high price of pain medications on the illegal drug market. Dr. Marc Fishman, who directs a treatment center in Maryland, says, "It becomes much cheaper and easier to sustain a habit with heroin." The resulting complications hurt patients, society, and health care payers alike.

For patients who want to stop using opioids, treatment for dependence or addiction is underused and under-available. For people who become dependent on opioids for back pain, the need can become critical. These are the kinds of treatment available to people like General Fridovich. But too many patients who want help in stopping opioids either can't find addiction treatment services or can't afford them.

We've seen the wide range of serious—and expensive—complications some of these patients experience. So better coverage of appropriate services may pay for itself in the long run.

While we're at it, we should ask about wider insurance coverage of treatments like chiropractic care and acupuncture. These are either not covered or have tight limitations in many insurance plans. The rationale is that expanding coverage would increase the volume of use and prove too expensive.

In part, this is because the treatments might be an add-on to conventional medical treatments rather than a substitute for them. Chiropractic care and acupuncture are labor-intensive and often involve multiple patient visits. People might abuse attractive services like massage therapy.

The counterargument from advocates is that these services are often safer than conventional drugs or surgery and may cost less in the end. Recent evidence-based guidelines suggest they offer benefits for people with persistent pain. Insurers could expand coverage without making it open-ended.

Our research group and others have tried to study whether people who use complementary and alternative medicine (CAM) actually incur higher health care costs. The study results are mixed. Some suggest higher costs, and some don't. That suggests it's a close call.

With Brook Martin again leading the charge, we examined national data from a household survey on health care use. We found that overall costs of care for back pain were no higher for patients who used CAM treatments than for those who used only conventional care. This was largely because people who used CAM were less likely to land in the hospital, thus offsetting costs of CAM therapy.

Among those who used CAM services for back pain, 75 percent used chiropractic care. The remainder was mostly for massage or acupuncture.

Of course, there's a risk of having people abuse more generous coverage. Who wouldn't go for several massages if insurance paid for them? Perhaps limited insurance coverage explains why CAM users in our study didn't incur higher costs. But it may be worth experimenting with more generous coverage schemes.

It remains to be seen if the Affordable Care Act (Obamacare) facilitates any of these proposals. But the needs described here are typical of many chronic diseases, not back pain alone. Insurance reform is essential if our health care system is going to serve those with chronic conditions as well as it serves those with acute injuries and illnesses.

Regulation of Drugs and Devices

The FDA is the key federal agency that regulates drugs and medical devices. It must approve new products, and it monitors manufacturing quality. One goal is to protect the public from the harm or expense of buying snake oil. But FDA approval often is not the "Good Housekeeping Seal of Approval" that we might hope for.

The agency faces constant criticism from industry. Drug and device makers claim the FDA drags its feet in approving new treatments that would benefit patients. Nonetheless, changes in funding and staffing in recent years have made the FDA faster to approve new drugs than agencies in most other countries.

That's a mistake, charge consumer safety advocates. They argue that rapid review doesn't leave time for discovering unusual complications or those resulting from long-term use of a product. They argue that it sets the bar too low for approving products. They also argue that the FDA fails to track patient results after approving new products.

Although the FDA gets criticized from many perspectives, we're all far better off with it than without it. But it lacks the authority, ability, and budget to do many of the things we might hope for.

As an example, the FDA doesn't require a new product to be any better than competing products already on the market. Or even just as good. The usual bar for a new drug is simply that it be better than a placebo. As a result, an FDA-approved drug can be better, worse, or the same as competing drugs that are often less expensive. And there are good examples of each of these possibilities. Remember the story of Vioxx, with greater side effects than previously available drugs and no indication of greater efficacy.

The bar for approving medical devices is even lower. The FDA approves the vast majority based on "substantial equivalence" to a product already on the market. Making this claim often doesn't even require doing tests in humans. Laboratory or animal tests often suffice.

The "substantial equivalence" mechanism is subjective, yet it accounts for the majority of new surgical implants and devices like TENS units. A former director of the entire FDA remarked, "New devices are less likely than drugs to have their safety established clinically before they are marketed." Considering the problems that occur with drugs like Vioxx, it's an alarming admission.

The FDA doesn't approve every possible use of a new product. A new drug or device is often approved for a narrow set of clinical conditions. But once it's approved for *something*, doctors can legally prescribe it for other purposes. As we saw with Neurontin and with Norian XR cement, manufacturers sometimes promote widespread use for conditions where any benefit is unproven.

The FDA doesn't approve TV or magazine ads for new drugs or devices before they're aired or printed. The agency does require that the ads be submitted for review, and fairly often requires changes. But potentially misleading ads can play for weeks or months before the FDA reviews them.

If a drug or device proves to be unsafe after it's already in use, the FDA can require a recall. But it generally doesn't recall products that simply turn out to be ineffective. The assumption is that market forces will handle that problem. But in fact, ineffective tests and treatments often are sold and used long after they've been disproven or found inferior to other products.

As one example, the painkiller Darvon was sold for fifty-three years, and was recalled from the market only in 2010. Over the years, several studies suggested it had only a minor effect on pain. It seemed to add no improvement over acetaminophen (Tylenol) alone. A review for postoperative pain suggested that ibuprofen was more effective. Yet Darvon was widely prescribed, and was withdrawn after decades of use only when studies found an increased risk of dangerous heart rhythms.

Finally, the FDA doesn't regulate surgical procedures at all, except for the devices used in surgery. But new surgical approaches or techniques don't receive any regulatory review.

These limitations have often resulted in new products that added little benefit but provided billions of dollars in profit for someone. Recall the stories of Neurontin for back pain or bone morphogenetic protein (BMP) for spinal fusion surgery.

With these problems in mind, we might want to encourage several reforms.

I like the idea of comparing competing products head-to-head and publicizing the results. This is something the government has shied away from, but it may be essential to improving medical outcomes and reducing costs.

A new research organization, the Patient Centered Outcomes Research Institute, may help to advance this idea. The Affordable Care Act created this public-private institute, which is just getting under way. The institute imposes rigorous scientific review on research proposals to ensure high quality.

I also like the idea of requiring randomized trials before approving any device that's going to be implanted in your body. This is the standard we require of drugs. It seems reasonable to expect that a product meant to be implanted permanently should be scrutinized as carefully as something that's just passing through.

I like restrictions on promoting off-label uses of drugs or devices. This is an existing rule. But it's one that the courts have recently begun to weaken, in the name of free speech. It seems that the courts have a different idea than scientists about the level of rigor needed to prove the efficacy and safety of new drugs. Without this safeguard, a return to the era of snake oil sales seems all too likely.

Tracking results of a new product after it hits the market is something the FDA has authority to do, but the agency admits it hasn't always done it well. The story of Vioxx comes to mind. The agency is moving toward more sophisticated strategies for "postmarketing surveillance," but it has a long way to go.

Specifically regarding opioid painkillers, some doctor groups have recently proposed more restrictive FDA labeling. A group called Physicians for Responsible Opioid Prescribing recently recommended that for non-cancer pain, opioid medications be labeled only for severe pain and not mild or moderate pain. The group also recommended limits on approved opioid doses, as a safeguard against the sixteen thousand annual fatal overdoses. The recommendations prompted controversy, with opposition from some organizations of pain doctors and pharmacy groups. On the other hand, the Drug Enforcement Agency supported the ideas.

As of late 2013, the FDA has moved to restrict the labeling of some painkillers as being for severe pain only. It has also recommended tighter prescribing controls on hydrocodone, the most frequently prescribed opioid. However, it chose not to recommend limits on dose or duration of use.

Technology Assessment

Most developed countries have an agency that rigorously reviews the scientific evidence on drugs and devices and then makes recommendations for insurance coverage. To some Americans, this smacks of rationing. But restricting access to things that don't work hardly seems like rationing. It's more like preventing snake oil sales, something most of us can support.

And most of us don't have the knowledge, time, or resources to access the scientific evidence, evaluate its quality, weigh various findings, and reach a valid conclusion about the efficacy and safety of every medical test or treatment. Especially when we're sick or in pain!

The FDA provides some of this kind of review. But we've seen the important limits on the agency's purview. We've seen that FDA approval of a drug or device is no indicator of whether the drug or device is any better or worse than competing treatments. And we've seen that there's no effort to regulate new surgical procedures or to compare surgical and nonsurgical treatments. So FDA approval tells us little about optimal treatment approaches.

Even if the information from a "technology assessment" agency weren't used to make insurance coverage decisions, it would help doctors and patients make better-informed clinical decisions.

We've experimented in the past with government agencies to conduct rigorous reviews of new medical technology. Some may remember the National Center for Health Care Technology. which briefly existed in the Carter administration. Or the Congressional Office of Technology Assessment, which had a longer life span.

These agencies were eliminated, in part because of vocal opposition from drug and device manufacturers. And remember the story of the Agency for Health Care Policy and Research that we discussed early on. It had a "near death" experience for writing guidelines on low back pain.

Because most other countries have a technology assessment agency, there are plenty of models to draw from. Britain's National Institute for

Clinical Excellence (NICE) is just one example. This agency produced the controversial British guidelines on low back pain that were critical of spinal injections.

There is a sad irony about turning to other countries for models to emulate. The irony is that most of those agencies were in turn modeled after our now-defunct Office of Technology Assessment.

What would it take for such an agency to succeed? It would take some major commitments and an ability to withstand the opposition that eliminated its predecessors. Dr. Jack Wennberg, a prominent doctor and policy researcher at Dartmouth Medical School, says this is what it would take: "The long view: stable funding; strong peer review to assure good science and freedom from conflicts of interest that affect judgments; policies that sustain the careers of leading scientists over a professional lifetime (keeping them free of dependency on funding from the drug and device companies whose products they evaluate); and deep commitment on the part of the scientific establishment, sufficient to withstand the wrath of practitioners and others with vested interests who find their favorite theories slain by evidence or demands for their services reduced because informed patients want less."

If we want better-quality and lower-cost medical care, an organization that provides medical technology assessment to inform our decisions would be most valuable. It would obviously be valuable for all medical tests and treatments, and not just those for back pain. But like the Federal Reserve in the banking industry, it would have to be relatively insulated from the vicissitudes of everyday politics.

The Media and Public Expectations

Government can't write policy that limits what the news media say. That's a free speech issue protected by the First Amendment. But the media can do a better job of policing themselves. It's tiring to see story after story about breakthroughs in back pain therapy while rates of chronic back pain and work disability continue to climb.

How about a moratorium on the word "breakthrough" in any story about back pain? Indeed, a prominent health journalist, Gary Schwitzer, proposes to ban this and some other words from health reporting in general. These include "cure," "miracle," "promising," and "dramatic."

Part of the problem is that many journalists feel pressure to exaggerate a bit if they want their stories on the front page or on the air. Another problem is that much of medical news comes from press releases, video mailings, and similar marketing materials produced by medical centers, drug companies, and device makers.

Schwitzer has plenty of other great recommendations for journalists, but I'll mention just one more here. Journalists should investigate links between researchers and sponsors who might benefit from new products or ideas the research supports. Those sponsors are often the manufacturers of a new product. And several studies show that research sponsored by drug or device makers is more positive toward their products than independent research.

But doctors and researchers share the blame, because they enjoy fame and attention like everyone else. Remember that one scientist likened being in the *New York Times* to winning a Nobel Prize. Media attention is good for both egos and future funding.

Of course, if it avoided marketing hype, the media could play a valuable role in educating the public. A government-sponsored public service campaign in Australia demonstrated the potential.

In the 1990s, the Australian state of Victoria found that back pain accounted for 50 percent of work disability claims, and the percentage was rising. Government officials and doctors worked with a public relations firm to develop a prime-time TV campaign of short "ads" featuring medical experts, sports stars, and entertainment personalities.

The messages emphasized continuing activity, avoiding bed rest, and caution in the use of imaging, medications, and surgery. A major theme was that there's a lot you can do to help yourself. The ads made good use of humor, personal experiences, and expert commentary.

Each ad included an endorsement from a relevant medical professional association. The campaign also included radio ads, billboards, and print publicity.

The results of the campaign were a 15 percent decline in back-related disability claims and a 20 percent decrease in medical costs per claim. Surveys showed a major shift in public views about rest, work loss, and the prognosis for recovery.

The program was also a stealth strategy for reeducating doctors, and surveys showed an improvement in their knowledge about back pain. All the improvements occurred in Victoria, but not in the adjacent state of New South Wales, where there was no similar media campaign. So the right media messages have a real potential for improving public health.

Promoting Shared Decision Making

It's hard to argue against helping to inform patients about decisions they face in the gray areas of medicine. And we've seen that there are plenty of gray areas in treating back pain. Studies suggest that the use of decision aids, like those we discussed earlier, is highly acceptable to both doctors and patients. Making decision aids more widely available seems like a good idea. But there are several barriers to doing it well.

Creating decision aids requires ample time, money, and expertise. It requires assembling the best scientific evidence, learning what patients' key concerns may be, and getting the advice of relevant specialists. It requires expertise in information technology and media to prepare a program that's attractive, easy to use, and easy to follow. It requires pilot testing, revisions, and a distribution strategy. Keeping programs up-to-date is a never-ending challenge.

And how do we ensure the integrity of these programs? It would be easy to lead patients to particular decisions, and that's actually the goal of marketing. The goal of a decision aid should be just the opposite— to lead the patient to his or her own best decision, not what's best for someone else's bottom line.

Furthermore, we're just learning how to integrate these programs into routine care. Should doctors' offices and hospitals maintain a library of programs? Should they be on the Internet? Formatted for your smartphone? How do we remind a doctor or patient—at just the right time—when a good decision aid is available?

If a doctor makes the effort to identify good decision aids and make them available, is he or she going to get paid for the time that takes?

These challenges suggest a role for policy, and some policy makers are stepping into the breach. The Affordable Care Act (Obamacare) authorized centers around the country to facilitate the creation, distribution, implementation, and updating of patient decision aids.

The law authorized the centers but didn't appropriate funds for them. So they're still an idea rather than a reality. If the idea has some appeal, Congress will need a push to fund it.

If decision aids become more widely available, it will be necessary to create a credentialing process for them. That is, someone will need to certify that a decision aid meets certain standards of accuracy, balance, and completeness before it becomes widely available. This would be a basic step toward building trust for the aids among doctors and patients. It would be analogous to FDA approval of drugs and devices, though we might hope for even higher standards.

Some states are already taking the initiative to encourage wider use of decision aids. In 2007, Washington State passed legislation that recognized shared decision making as a particularly high standard of informed consent. It also required demonstration projects and succeeded in winning the support of the Washington State Medical Association.

One of the early demonstrations, at the Group Health Cooperative of Puget Sound, showed that patient enthusiasm was high, and the health plan saved money. For example, one part of the project focused on hip and knee replacement surgery. These are operations where no single decision is right for everyone. As a result, the choices are highly sensitive to both patient and doctor preferences. With the use of decision aids, rates of knee replacement surgery fell 38 percent.

Ultimately, some advocates imagine that "decision quality" would become a measure of quality of care. A health plan could measure decision quality, for example, by assessing patient knowledge about the decision and ratings of involvement in decision making. A more ambitious approach might even assess the congruence of a decision with the patient's stated values.

Funding Research

Like Rodney Dangerfield, back pain "don't get no respect." In the push and shove of priorities for funding medical research, things like cancer and heart disease always win. Those diseases are potentially fatal, after all, and back pain rarely is. But the impact of back pain on quality of life, work disability, and costs of both medical care and disability compensation makes it a huge burden.

Back pain deserves a higher priority in the research funding sweepstakes. Unfortunately, we're in an era when government support for research is shrinking rather than expanding.

And industry is unlikely to support research that could run counter to its own financial interests. Industry-supported research will inevitably focus on gaining regulatory approval and advancing marketing aims rather than answering the questions most important to patients and doctors.

Those are such questions as, What's the balance of benefits and risks? Which treatment approach works best? What sequences or combinations of treatments are most effective? How can we help patients make the best decisions for themselves? How do we support beneficial lifestyle changes?

One newer approach to research funding involves insurance carriers, including both government and private carriers. At least in theory, insurers have an interest in paying for things that work and avoiding things that don't. The approach is called coverage with evidence development (CED), and it goes something like this.

Insurers often pay for treatments that have little scientific support, just because they've become a standard of care. In fact, they risk lawsuits if they refuse coverage for things that doctors and patients have come to expect. We've discussed several examples of common back pain treatments for which the scientific evidence is weak or nonexistent.

With CED, an insurer might determine that there's too little evidence about efficacy or safety to continue paying for a treatment without getting better data. The insurer might then decide to pay for the treatment only if patients and doctors agree to participate in a clinical trial to get that data.

This strategy was used by Medicare with great success in testing a new surgical treatment for emphysema. Despite great enthusiasm among surgeons, the operation proved to be useless or harmful for all but a tiny handful of patients. The resulting limits on its use created enormous savings for Medicare, which allowed better coverage of effective treatments.

Recall the controversy about transcutaneous electrical nerve stimulation for treating back pain, which we discussed at the beginning of this book. Recall too that Medicare recently decided on a CED approach to further funding for that particular form of treatment. This may prove to be an important new strategy for funding research on back pain.

Given the uncertainties about many back pain treatments, and the high stakes, I hope people with back pain will embrace the notion of more and better research. And I hope they'll be willing to participate in it.

That requires not insisting on a new treatment just because it's new. It requires a more skeptical attitude, realizing that newer isn't necessarily better. We should remember the stories of Norian XR cement, Vioxx, and BMP as cautionary tales.

It means not assuming that newer is better. It means reserving judgment and participating in clinical trials. While this may be frustrating, I believe it's the only way out of some of the holes we find ourselves in.

You may recognize that many of the policy suggestions here are relevant to areas of medicine well beyond back pain. Indeed, back pain exemplifies many problems with our larger health care system.

Conclusions

Dr. Donald Berwick is a former head of Medicare and an energetic advocate for improving the quality of care. He's fond of pointing out that every system is perfectly designed to get the results that it gets. If our health care system generates high costs, promotes ineffective care, and creates avoidable complications, it's because we've inadvertently designed the system to get exactly those results.

In care for back pain, we do this by performing tests when they're unlikely to help and responding to alarming but meaningless results. We do it by prescribing medications and procedures with proven risks but unproven benefits. We do it by expecting a quick fix from a probe, a pill, or a procedure when real benefits require harder lifestyle changes. We do it with unrealistic expectations of a pain-free life. We do it by responding to financial incentives for more rather than better care. And we do it by ignoring and underfunding the treatments that appear to be most helpful.

For back pain, here are the results: steadily increasing use of imaging tests, opioids, injections, and surgery. Costs that are rising faster than the rest of medical care. And at a population level, worsening patient function and work disability. We've perfectly designed our health care system to produce these results.

It's easier to understand this situation if you remember that the back business is indeed a business. This is the story of too much medical care today. In a for-profit health care system, the first concern is the bottom line rather than the patient's welfare. And too often it follows a business ethos: *caveat emptor*—buyer beware.

Much of the needed change will come from empowering patients and the public. Better information will produce better choices. Better

self-care will reduce the need for medical intervention. Reducing unnecessary procedures will reduce avoidable complications. Greater
physical activity will result in not only less heart disease and cancer in
the future but less back pain today.

We can do better. But you'll have to insist.

NOTES

1. Back Pain Nation

1 *"Two-thirds of adults report back pain at some time in their lives"*: R. C. Lawrence, D. T. Felson, C. G. Helmick, L. M. Arnold, H. Choi, and R. A. Deyo, et al., Estimates of the prevalence of arthritis and other rheumatic conditions in the United States: Part II, *Arthritis Rheum* 58 (2008): 26–35.

1 *"When our research team at the University of Washington scrutinized"*: R. A. Deyo, S. K. Mirza, J. A. Turner, and B. I. Martin, Overtreating chronic back pain: Time to back off?, *J Am Board Fam Med* 22 (2009): 62–68.

2 *"Our research group's best estimate, based on national surveys: $86 billion in 2005"*: B. I. Martin, R. A. Deyo, S. K. Mirza, J. A. Turner, B. A. Comstock, W. Hollingworth, and S. D. Sullivan, Expenditures and health status among adults with back and neck problems, *JAMA* 299 (2008): 656–664.

2 *"Market watchers estimate that spinal implants alone"*: Market Research. com, Spinal implants—global pipeline analysis, opportunity assessment and market forecasts to 2016, October 15, 2010, http://www.marketrese arch.com/GlobalData-v3648/Spinal-Implants-Global-Pipeline-Opportu nity-2840291/.

2 *"The national hospital bill for those operations"*: HCUPnet, Agency for Healthcare Research and Quality, http://hcupnet.ahrq.gov/HCUPnet.jsp.

2 *"Drug market analysts estimated the market for narcotic painkillers"*: J. Fauber, Chronic pain fuels boom in opioids, *MedPage Today*, February 19, 2012, http:// www.medpagetoday.com/Neurology/PainManagement/31254.

2   *"Our rate of back surgery"*: D. C. Cherkin, R. A. Deyo, J. D. Loeser, T. Bush, and G. Waddell, An international comparison of back surgery rates, *Spine* 19 (1994): 1201–1206.

2   *"Americans seem to have a unique conviction"*: M. Kim, R. J. Blendon, and B. M. Benson, How interested are Americans in new medical technologies? A multicountry comparison, *Health Aff (Millwood)* 20 (2001): 194–201.

4   *"David Freedman, a science and business journalist"*: D. H. Freedman, *Wrong: Why Experts Keep Failing Us—and How to Know When Not to Trust Them* (New York: Little, Brown, 2010).

6   *"Other readers will question the motives"*: S. H. Woolf, The price of false beliefs: Unrealistic expectations as a contributor to the health care crisis, *Ann Fam Med* 10 (2012): 491–494.

7   *"Annual surveys of people with back pain"*: Martin et al., Expenditures and health status among adults.

7   *"Work disability due to back pain has been increasing"*: Deyo, Overtreating chronic back pain.

7   *"And rates of repeat surgery have been going up instead of down"*: B. I. Martin, S. K. Mirza, B. A. Comstock, D. T. Gray, W. Kreuter, and R. A. Deyo, Are lumbar spine reoperation rates falling with greater use of fusion surgery and new surgical technology? *Spine* 32 (2007): 2119–2126.

7   *"First, research shows that most people with a recent onset"*: J. Coste, G. Delecoeuillerie, and A. Cohen de Lara, et al., Clinical course and prognostic factors in acute low back pain: An inception cohort study in primary care practice, *Br Med J* 308 (1994): 577–580; J. Coste, G. Lefrancois, and F. Guillemin, et al., Prognosis and quality of life in patients with acute low back pain: Insights from a comprehensive inception cohort study, *Arthritis Rheum* 51 (2004): 168–176.

7   *"The overabundance of cures, and variations in clinical practice"*: D. C. Cherkin, R. A. Deyo, K. Wheeler, and M. A. Ciol, Physician variation in diagnostic testing for low back pain: Who you see is what you get, *Arthritis Rheum* 37 (1994): 15–22.

8   *"A New York pain specialist, Dr. Seth Waldman"*: J. Groopman, A knife in the back, *New Yorker*, April 8, 2002.

8   *"In a recent review, he and his colleagues counted more than two hundred available treatment options"*: S. Haldeman and S. Dagenais, A supermarket approach to the evidence-informed management of chronic low back pain, *Spine J* 8 (2008): 1–7.

9   *"Pronovost argues that we have two American health care systems"*: P. J. Pronovost and M. L. Weisfeldt, Science-based training in patient safety and quality, *Ann Intern Med* 157 (2012): 141–143.

9   *"As a medical editor reminds us, once an industry builds up"*: J. O. Neher, Reason and reversal, *Evidence-Based Practice* 16, no. 8 (2013): 3.

11   *"And there was research using large-bore needles"*: A. L. Nachemson, The lumbar spine: An orthopedic challenge, *Spine* 1 (1976): 59–71.

11   *"We would take patients from a walk-in clinic"*: R. A. Deyo, A. K. Diehl, and M. Rosenthal, How many days of bed rest for acute low back pain? A randomized clinical trial, *N Engl J Med* 315 (1986): 1064–1070.

13   *"Patients in both the true TENS and the sham TENS groups improved"*: R. A. Deyo, N. E. Walsh, D. C. Martin, L. S. Schoenfeld, and S. Ramamurthy, A controlled trial of transcutaneous electrical nerve stimulation (TENS) and exercise for chronic low back pain, *N Engl J Med* 322 (1990): 1627–1634.

13   *"Remember, Scott Haldeman identified two hundred different treatments"*: Haldeman and Dagenais, Supermarket approach.

14   *"Nonetheless, a recent review of research studies"*: A. Khadlikar, D. O. Odebiyi, L. Brosseau, and G. A. Wells, Transcutaneous electrical nerve stimulation (TENS) versus placebo for chronic low-back pain, *Cochrane Database of Systematic Reviews*, issue 4 (2008), art. no. CD003008, doi:10.1002/14651858. CD003008.pub3.

14   *"Guidelines from the American Academy of Neurology"*: R. M. Dubinsky and J. Miyasaki, Assessment: Efficacy of transcutaneous electric nerve stimulation in the treatment of pain in neurologic disorders (an evidence-based review); Report of the Therapeutics and Technology Assessment Subcommittee of the American Academy of Neurology, *Neurology* 74 (2010): 173–176.

14   *"Medicare officials have taken the stance"*: Department of Health and Human Services, Centers for Medicare and Medicaid Services, Transcutaneous electrical nerve stimulation (TENS) for chronic low back pain (CLBP), *MLN Matters,* no. MM7836, Dec. 4, 2012, http://www.cms.gov/ Outreach-and-Education/Medicare-Learning-Network-MLN/MLNMat tersArticles/downloads/MM7836.pdf.

16   *"The research and guideline efforts were simply too much"*: R. A. Deyo, B. M. Psaty, G. Simon, E. H. Wagner, and G. S. Omenn, The messenger under attack—intimidation of researchers by special-interest groups, *N Engl J Med* 336 (1997): 1176–1180.

16   *"The Agency for Health Care Policy and Research became a political target"*: B. H. Gray, M. K. Gusmano, and S. R. Collins, AHCPR and the changing politics of health services research, *Health Aff (Millwood)* 2003 (Jan–Jun), Suppl Web Exclusives: W3-283–307.

16   *"The North American Spine Society later faced allegations"*: G. Borzo, Societies caught in fraud cases: Product liability lawsuits raise questions about CME vs. promotion, *American Medical News* 40, no. 18 (1997): 1, 24.

17   *"AcroMed, which had subpoenaed our research records, settled thousands of patient lawsuits"*: R. F. Heary, Pedicle screw controversy, Spine Section Newsletter, American Association of Neurological Surgeons and Congress of

Neurological Surgeons, September 1997, http://www.spinesection.org/files/pdfs/newsletters/spinenews0997.pdf.

17 *"Years later, in 2006, Sofamor Danek's parent company, Medtronic"*: R. Abelson, Medtronic will settle accusations on kickbacks, *New York Times*, July 19, 2006.

17 *"Also in 2006, the successor to the Agency for Health Care Policy and Research"*: D. C. McCrory, D. A. Turner, M. B. Patwardhan, and W. J. Richardson, *Spinal Fusion for Degenerative Disease Affecting the Lumbar Spine* (Draft Evidence Report) (Baltimore: Centers for Medicare and Medicaid Services, 2006), http://www.cms.hhs.gov/determinationprocess/downloads/id41ta.pdf.

17 *"According to government statistics, spinal fusion surgery"*: HCUPnet, Agency for Healthcare Research and Quality, http://hcupnet.ahrq.gov/HCUP net.jsp.

17 *"Dr. Edward Benzel, a neurosurgeon at the prestigious Cleveland Clinic"*: R. Abelson and M. Petersen, An operation to ease back pain bolsters the bottom line, too, *New York Times*, December 31, 2003.

2. Even the Best and Brightest

20 *"We now have details of Kennedy's back problems"*: Kennedy's back pain history was compiled from the following sources: R. Dallek, *An Unfinished Life: John F. Kennedy, 1917–1963* (New York: Little, Brown, 2003); R. Dallek, The medical ordeals of JFK, *Atlantic*, December 2002; R. A. Hart, Failed spine surgery syndrome in the life and career of John Fitzgerald Kennedy, *J Bone Joint Surg Am* 88-A (2006): 1141–1148; R. J. Donovan, *PT 109: John F. Kennedy in World War II* (Greenwich, Conn.: Fawcett, 1961).

22 *"After reviewing the records, my orthopedist colleague"*: A. Dworkin, OHSU surgeon delves into back story on JFK's back, *Oregonian*, September 29, 2006.

25 *"Kraus was an Austrian immigrant"*: Obituary: Dr. Hans Kraus, 90, originator of sports medicine in U.S., dies, *New York Times*, March 7, 1996.

25 *"Records in the Kennedy Library show that Kraus examined JFK"*: Records of Dr. Hans Kraus, John F. Kennedy Presidential Library and Museum, Boston, MA.

25 *"A* New York Times *article in December 1961 noted"*: President's back reported better, *New York Times*, December 14, 1961.

26 *"Later press reports were even more admiring"*: D. Wise, The White House. *New York Herald Tribune*, July 1962.

26 *"Following Kennedy's assassination, Admiral Burkley wrote to thank Kraus"*: Records of Dr. Hans Kraus, John F. Kennedy Presidential Library and Museum, Boston, MA.

26 *"Evelyn Lincoln, Kennedy's long-time assistant, wrote to Kraus years later"*: Records of Dr. Hans Kraus, John F. Kennedy Presidential Library and Museum, Boston, MA.

3. What's Wrong? What's Not? Can We Tell the Difference?

31 *"So why do the clinical guidelines from eleven countries"*: B. W. Koes, M. W. van Tulder, R. Ostelo, A. K. Burton, and G. Waddell, Clinical guidelines for the management of low back pain in primary care: An international comparison, *Spine* 26 (2001): 2504–2514.

32 *"And why do U.S. guidelines recommend"*: R. Chou, A. Qaseem, D. K. Owens, and P. Shekelle, Clinical Guidelines Committee of the American College of Physicians, Diagnostic imaging for low back pain: Advice for high-value health care from the American College of Physicians. *Ann Intern Med* 154 (2011): 181–189.

33 *"Glands like the adrenal gland and the pituitary gland can show nodules on MRI"*: M. E. Molitch and E. J. Russell, The pituitary "incidentaloma," *Ann Intern Med* 112 (1990): 925–931; M. M. Grumbach, B. M. Biller, and G. D. Braunstein, Management of the clinically inapparent adrenal mass ("incidentaloma"), *Ann Intern Med* 138 (2003): 424–429.

33 *"Dr. Boden managed to find sixty-seven adults"*: S. D. Boden, D. O. David, and T. S. Dina, et al., Abnormal magnetic-resonance scans of the lumbar spine in asymptomatic subjects, *J Bone Joint Surg Am* 72 (1990): 403–408.

34 *"That is to say, identical twins have very similar-looking spines"*: M. C. Battie and T. Videman, Lumbar disc degeneration: Epidemiology and genetics, *J Bone Joint Surg Am* 88-A, Suppl 2 (2006): 3–9.

35 *"But this study has been replicated about a dozen times"*: R. A. Deyo and J. N. Weinstein, Low back pain, *N Engl J Med* 344 (2001): 363–370; J. J. Jarvik, W. Hollingworth, P. Heagerty, D. R. Haynor, and R. A. Deyo, The Longitudinal Assessment of Imaging and Disability of the Back (LAIDBack) Study: Baseline data, *Spine* 26, no. 10 (2001): 1158–1166.

35 *"You might also ask, what about CT scans or other imaging tests?"*: S. W. Wiesel, N. Tsourmas, and H. L. Feffer, et al., 1984 Volvo Award in Clinical Sciences, A study of computer-assisted tomography, I: The incidence of positive CAT scans in an asymptomatic group of patients, *Spine* 9 (1984): 549–551.

35 *"If we look at herniated discs"*: A. Bozzao, M. Gallucci, and C. Masciocchi, et al., Lumbar disc herniation: MR imaging assessment of natural history in patients treated without surgery, *Radiology* 185 (1992): 135–141; M.-C. Delauche-Cavallier, C. Buder, and J.-D. Laredo, et al., Lumbar disc herniation: Computed tomography scan changes after conservative treatment of nerve root compression, *Spine* 17 (1992): 927–933.

35   *"Dr. Jarvik led our Seattle research team in a study similar to Boden's"*:
J. G. Jarvik, W. Hollingworth, P. J. Heagerty, D. R. Haynor, E. J. Boyko,
and R. A. Deyo, Three-year incidence of low back pain in an initially asymptomatic cohort: Clinical and imaging risk factors, *Spine* 30 (2005):
1541–1548.

36   *"A British study enrolled people with back pain who had no sign of underlying
infection"*: D. Kendrick, K. Fielding, and E. Bentley, et al., Radiography of
the lumbar spine in primary care patients with low back pain: Randomized
controlled trial, *Br Med J* 322, no. 7283 (2001): 400–405.

37   *"Another study, done at the Cleveland Clinic, did MRI scans"*: L. M. Ash, M.
T. Modic, and N. A. Obuchowski, et al., Effects of diagnostic information,
per se, on patient outcomes in acute radiculopathy and low back pain, *AJNR
Am J Neuroradiol* 29 (2008): 1098–1103.

37   *"Several years ago, we did a study that showed"*: J. G. Jarvik, W. Hollingworth, and B. Martin, et al., Rapid magnetic resonance imaging vs radio-
graphs for patients with low back pain: A randomized controlled trial, *JAMA*
289 (2003): 2810–2818.

38   *"And where the rates of spine imaging are the highest"*: J. D. Lurie, N. J. Birk-
meyer, and J. N. Weinstein, Rates of advanced spinal imaging and spine
surgery, *Spine* 28 (2003): 616–620.

38   *"When we examined Medicare claims, we found an increase of 307 percent"*:
R. A. Deyo, S. K. Mirza, J. A. Turner, and B. I. Martin, Overtreating chronic
back pain: Time to back off? *J Am Board Fam Med* 22 (2009): 62–68.

38   *"American College of Physicians and a group of family doctors"*: Good Stew-
ardship Working Group, The "Top 5" lists in primary care: Meeting the
responsibility of professionalism, *Arch Intern Med* 171 (2011): 1385–1390.

4. Painkillers: Easy Solutions Sometimes Aren't

41   *"I earlier described David Fridovich as a tough guy"*: Background on General David Fridovich was compiled from the following sources: A. Colindres, Compelled to lead: David Fridovich's story of painkillers, football,
and leadership, *Knox College Magazine*, Spring 2013, http://www.knox.edu/
alumni-and-friends/knox-magazine-and-more/spring-2013/compelled-to-
lead.html; We are Knox . . . David Fridovich '74, Three-Star Lieutenant
General, Knox College Trustee, 2007 Alumni Achievement Award winner,
http://www.knox.edu/profile-index/alumni-and-friends/fridovich-david-
74.html; 2007 Alumni Achievement Awards, David P. Fridovich '74, 2007
Alumni Achievement Award recipient for his service in the Armed Forces,
http://www.knox.edu/alumni-and-friends/alumni-awards/alumni-achi
evement-awards/2007-alumni-achievement-awards.html; Lt. Gen. David P.

Fridovich '74 retires after 37 years of military service, November 18, 2011, http://www.knox.edu/news-and-events/news-archive/lt-general-david-fridovich-74-retires.html.

43 *"General Fridovich's back pain began between trips to war zones"*: Information on the general's back pain was compiled from these sources in addition to those above: G. Zoroya, General's story a warning about use of painkillers, *USA Today*, January 27, 2011, http://usatoday30.usatoday.com/news/military/2011-01-27-1Adruggeneral27_CV_N.htm; G. Zoroya, Up to 35% of wounded soldiers addicted to drugs, *USA Today*, January 26, 2011, http://usatoday30.usatoday.com/news/military/2011-01-26-sol dieraddicts26_ST_N.htm; personal interview, November 23, 2012.

47 *"Cindy McCain, the wife of Senator John McCain"*: K. Kindy, A tangled story of addiction: Consequences of Cindy McCain's drug abuse were more complex than she has portrayed, *Washington Post*, September 12, 2008.

47 *"Other people develop a paradoxical* increase *in pain sensitivity"*: J. Mao, Opioid-induced abnormal pain sensitivity: Implications in clinical opioid therapy, *Pain* 100 (2002): 213–217; L. F. Chu, M. S. Angst, and D. Clark, Opioid-induced hyperalgesia in humans: Molecular mechanisms and clinical considerations, *Clin J Pain* 24 (2008): 479–495.

48 *"For example, among patients who had a spinal fusion operation"*: S. Blumenthal, P. C. McAfee, and R. D. Guyer, et al., A prospective, randomized, multicenter Food and Drug Administration investigational device exemptions study of lumbar total disc replacement with the CHARITE artificial disc versus lumbar fusion, Part I: Evaluation of clinical outcomes, *Spine* 30 (2005): 1565–1575.

5. Painkillers and the Marketing of Pain

51 *"Sales of prescription opioids quadrupled between 1999 and 2010"*: L. J. Paulozzi, C. M. Jones, K. A. Mack, and R. A. Rudd, Vital signs: Overdoses of prescription opioid pain relievers, United States, 1999–2008, *MMWR Morb Mortal Wkly Rep* 60 (2011): 1487–1492.

51 *"Instead, doctors most often prescribe opioids for problems like back pain and arthritis"*: T. J. Hudson, M. J. Edlund, D. E. Steffick, S. P. Tripathi, and M. D. Sullivan, Epidemiology of regular prescribed opioid use: Results from a national, population-based survey, *J Pain Sympt Mgmt* 36 (2008): 280–288; D. Boudreau, M. Von Korff, and C. M. Rutter, et al., Trends in long-term opioid therapy for chronic non-cancer pain, *Pharmacoepidemiol Drug Safety* 18 (2009): 1166–1175.

51 *"And the largest quantity of opioids go to people with long-term pain"*: M. Von Korff, A. Kolodny, R. A. Deyo, and R. Chou, Long-term opioid therapy reconsidered, *Ann Intern Med* 155 (2011): 325–328.

51   *"But more than half the patients who regularly use prescription opioids
      have back pain"*: Hudson et al., Epidemiology of regular prescribed opi-
      oid use.

51   *"Here the benefits are far less clear, the doses often higher"*: B. J. Morasco, J.
      P. Duckart, T. P. Carr, R. A. Deyo, and S. K. Dobscha, Clinical charac-
      teristics of veterans prescribed high doses of opioid medications for chronic
      non-cancer pain, *Pain* 151 (2010): 625–632; A. Deshpande, A. D. Fur-
      lan, A. Mailis-Gagnon, S. Atlas, and D. Turk, Opioids for chronic low-
      back pain, *Cochrane Database of Systematic Reviews*, issue 3 (2007), art. no.
      CD004959. doi:10.1002/14651858.CD004959.pub3; B. Meier, Pain pills
      add cost and delays to job injuries, *New York Times*, June 2, 2012.

52   *"Even these studies tracked patients for only four months or less"*: B. A. Mar-
      tell, P. G. O'Connor, R. D. Kerns, W. C. Becker, K. H. Morales, and T. R.
      Kosten, et al., Systematic review: Opioid treatment for chronic back pain;
      Prevalence, efficacy, and association with addiction, *Ann Intern Med* 146
      (2007): 116–127.

52   *"Surveys show that patients who take long-term opioids actually report worse
      pain"*: J. Eriksen, P. Sjogren, E. Bruera, O. Ekholm, and N. K. Rasmussen,
      Critical issues on opioids in chronic non-cancer pain: An epidemiological
      study, *Pain* 125 (2006): 172–179.

52   *"But new studies are showing that large doses of opioids increase the risk of over-
      dose and death"*: A. S. B. Bohnert, M. V. Valenstein, M. J. Bair, D. Gano-
      czy, J. F. McCarthy, and M. A. Ilgen, et al., Association between opioid
      prescribing patterns and opioid overdose-related deaths, *JAMA* 305 (2011):
      1315–1321; Von Korff et al., Long-term opioid therapy reconsidered.

52   *"Opioid-related deaths have quadrupled since 1999"*: Paulozzi et al., Vital
      signs.

52   *"That meant 16,651 deaths in 2010 alone"*: C. M. Jones, K. A. Mack, and L.
      J. Paulozzi, Pharmaceutical overdose deaths, United States, 2010, *JAMA* 309
      (2013): 657–659.

52   *"At age twenty-eight, Steve Rummler had back and leg pain"*: M. Newfield,
      Prescription drug deaths: Two stories, CNN, November 15, 2012, http://
      www.cnn.com/2012/11/15/health/deadly-dose-jackson-rummler.

53   *"Along with mortality, admissions to substance abuse treatment have in-
      creased 400 percent"*: S. Okie, A flood of opioids, a rising tide of deaths,
      N Engl J Med 363 (2010): 1981–1985.

53   *"The White House Office of Drug Control Policy describes the current situa-
      tion"*: Office of National Drug Control Policy, Epidemic: Responding to
      America's prescription drug abuse crisis, 2011, http://www.whitehouse.gov/
      sites/default/files/ondcp/policy-and-research/rx_abuse_plan.pdf.

53   *"Studies of older adults show decreased short-term memory"*: P. Sjogren, A. B.
      Thomsen, and A. K. Olsen, Impaired neuropsychological performance in

chronic nonmalignant pain patients receiving long-term oral opioid therapy, *J Pain Sympt Mgmt* 19 (2000): 100–108.

53 *"Many people don't realize that long-term opioid use can lead to sexual problems"*: H. W. Daniell, Hypogonadism in men consuming sustained-action oral opioids, *J Pain* 3 (2002): 377–384; H. W. Daniell, Opioid endocrinopathy in women consuming prescribed sustained-action opioids for control of nonmalignant pain, *J Pain* 9 (2008): 28–36; R. A. Deyo, D. H. Smith, and E. S. Johnson, et al., Prescription opioids for back pain and use of medications for erectile dysfunction, *Spine* 38 (2013): 909–915.

53 *"In older adults, opioid therapy increases falls, fractures, and osteoporosis"*: K. W. Saunders, K. M. Dunn, J. O. Merrill, M. Sullivan, C. Weisner, J. B. Braden, B. M. Psaty, and M. Von Korff, Relationship of opioid use and dosage levels to fractures in older chronic pain patients, *J Gen Intern Med* 25 (2010): 310–315; A. Grey, K. Rix-Trott, A. Horne, G. Gamble, M. Bolland, and I. R. Reid, Decreased bone density in men on methadone maintenance therapy, *Addiction* 106 (2011): 349–354; L. Rolita, A. Spegman, X. Tang, and B. N. Cronstein, Greater number of narcotic analgesic prescriptions for osteoarthritis is associated with falls and fractures in elderly adults, *J Am Geriatr Soc* 61 (2013): 335–340.

54 *"Dr. Ballantyne is an outspoken critic of the way doctors currently prescribe opioids"*: J. C. Ballantyne, Pain medicine: Repairing a fractured dream, *Anesthesiology* 114 (2011): 243–246.

54 *"In 2011, the market for prescription opioids was $8.4 billion"*: J. Fauber, Chronic pain fuels boom in opioids, *MedPage Today*, February 19, 2012, http://www.medpagetoday.com/Neurology/PainManagement/31254.

54 *"And the single most prescribed drug in the United States is hydrocodone"*: D. J. DeNoon, The 10 most prescribed drugs: Most-prescribed drug list differs from list of drugs with biggest market share, *WebMD Health News*, April 20, 2011, http://www.webmd.com/news/20110420/the-10-most-prescribed-drugs.

54 *"American Academy of Pain Medicine (AAPM), lists members"*: American Academy of Pain Medicine, Corporate Relations Council Profiles, http://www.painmed.org/membercenter/corporate-relations-council-profiles/.

55 *"The same companies appear as Corporate Council Members"*: American Pain Society, Corporate Council Members http://www.americanpainsociety.org/support-aps/content/corporate-council-members.html.

55 *"Senate Finance Committee announced an investigation"*: Baucus, Grassley seek answers about opioid manufacturers' ties to medical groups, U.S. Senate Committee on Finance, May 8, 2012, http://www.finance.senate.gov/newsroom/chairman/release/?id=021c94cd-b93e-4e4e-bcf4-7f4b9fae0047.

55 *"American Academy of Pain Medicine received $1.3 million"*: J. Fauber, Chronic pain fuels boom in opioids.

56 *"For example, a 2003 report from the General Accounting Office"*: General Accounting Office, Prescription drugs: OxyContin abuse and diversion and efforts to address the problem, December 2003, report no. GAO-04-110), http://www.gao.gov/new.items/d04110.pdf.

56 *"In addition, the American Pain Society and the Joint Commission"*: C. L. Fernandes, Practitioner Forum: The fifth vital sign, *Federal Practitioner*, December 2010, 26–28; P. Lanser and S. Gesell, Pain management: The fifth vital sign, *Healthc Benchmarks* 8, no. 6 (2001): 68–70, 62.

56 *"Doctors today often have part of their incomes tied to patient satisfaction"*: A. Lembke, Why doctors prescribe opioids to known opioid abusers, *N Engl J Med* 367 (2012): 1580–1581.

56 *"In 1996, the year of OxyContin's debut"*: Von Korff et al., Long-term opioid therapy reconsidered.

57 *"A decade later, Purdue Pharma's top three executives pled guilty"*: B. Meier, In guilty plea, OxyContin maker to pay $600 million, *New York Times*, May 10, 2007.

57 *"In 2008, Cephalon reached a settlement"*: Fauber, Chronic pain fuels boom in opioids.

57 *"But no one conveyed the message"*: L. E. Chaparro, A. D. Furlan, A. Deshpande, A. Mailis-Gagnon, S. Atlas, and D. C. Turk, Opioids compared to placebo or other treatments for chronic low-back pain, *Cochrane Database of Systematic Reviews*, , issue 8 (2013), art. no. CD004959, doi:10.1002/14651858. CD004959.pub4.

57 *"How much effect does prescription painkiller abuse have on our society?"*: H. G. Birnbaum, A. G. White, M. Schiller, T. Waldman, J. M. Cleveland, and Cl. Roland, Societal costs of prescription opioid abuse, dependence, and misuse in the United States, *Pain Medicine* 12 (2011): 657–667.

58 *"In retrospect, one vocal doctor argued"*: A. Kolodny, Opioids are rarely the answer, Room for Debate, *New York Times*, February 16, 2012. http://www.nytimes.com/roomfordebate/2012/02/15/how-to-curb-prescription-drug-abuse/opioids-are-rarely-the-answer.

58 *"Others have recently summarized that there's little evidence"*: D. N. Juurlink, I. A. Dhalla, and L. S. Nelson, Improving opioid prescribing: The New York City recommendations, *JAMA* 309 (2013): 879–880.

6. Pain Management, Now That's Money

59 *"An FDA scientist estimated that Vioxx caused"*: D. M. Graham, D. Campen, and R. Hull, et al., Risk of acute myocardial infarction and sudden cardiac death in patients treated with cyclo-oxygenase 2 selective and non-selective non-steroidal anti-inflammatory drugs: Nested case-control study, *Lancet* 365 (2005): 475–481.

59   *"Several studies combined showed that the risk"*: P. Juni, L. Nartey, and S. Reichenback, et al., Risk of cardiovascular events and rofecoxib: Cumulative meta-analysis, *Lancet* 364 (2004): 2021–2029; J. S. Ross, D. Madigan, and K. P. Hill, et al., Pooled analysis of rofecoxib placebo-controlled clinical trial data: Lessons for postmarket pharmaceutical safety surveillance, *Arch Intern Med* 169 (2009): 1976–1984.

59   *"Other researchers found that most who took Vioxx"*: C. Dai, R. S. Stafford, and G. C. Alexander, National trends in cyclooxygenase-2 inhibitor use since market release: Nonselective diffusion of a selectively cost-effective innovation, *Arch Intern Med* 165 (2005): 171–177.

60   *"In 2007, Merck settled 26,000 cases for almost $5 billion"*: F. Charatan, Merck to pay $5bn in rofecoxib claims, *Brit Med J* 335 (2007): 1011; F. Charatan, Merck to pay $58 m in settlements of rofecoxib advertising, *Brit Med J* 336 (2008): 1208–1209; J. H. Tanne, Merck pays $1bn penalty in relation to promotion of rofecoxib, *Br Med J* 343 (2011): d7702.

60   *"To this end, the company paid for scientific articles to be ghostwritten"*: J. S. Ross, K. P. Hill, D. S. Egilman, and H. M. Krumholz, Guest authorship and ghostwriting in publications related to rofecoxib: A case study of industry documents from rofecoxib litigation, *JAMA* 299 (2008): 1800–1812.

60   *"It undertook so-called seeding trials"*: K. P. Hill, J. S. Ross, D. S. Egilman, and H. M. Krumholz, The ADVANTAGE seeding trial: A review of internal documents, *Ann Int Med* 149 (2008): 251–258.

60   *"The story of Dr. Gurkipal Singh"*: S. Prakash, Part 1: Documents suggest Merck tried to censor Vioxx critics, National Public Radio, June 9, 2005, transcript at http://www.npr.org/templates/story/story.php?storyId= 4696609; S. Prakash, Part 2: Did Merck try to censor Vioxx critics? National Public Radio, June 9, 2005, transcript at http://www.npr.org/templates/ story/story.php?storyId=4696711; S. Prakash, Merck attempted to quash Vioxx criticism, National Public Radio, June 10, 2005, transcript at http:// www.npr.org/templates/story/story.php?storyId=4697507.

62   *"A young biologist, Dr. David Franklin"*: C. S. Landefeld and M. Steinman, The Neurontin legacy—marketing through misinformation and manipulation, *N Engl J Med* 360 (2009): 103–106.

62   *"The federal suit that followed the whistleblower suit alleged"*: compiled from M. Petersen, Whistle-blower says marketers broke the rules to push a drug, *New York Times*, March 14, 2002, p. C1; M. Petersen, Doctor explains why he blew the whistle, *New York Times*, March 13, 2003, p. C1; M. Petersen, Suit says company promoted drug in exam rooms, *New York Times*, May 15, 2002, p. C1.

62   *"Court documents described a memo to Parke-Davis sales representatives"*: L. Kowalczyk, Drug company push on doctors disclosed, *Boston Globe*, May 19, 2002, p. A1; M. Petersen, Court papers suggest scale of drug's use, *New York Times*, May 30, 2003, p. C1.

63 *"Internal documents show that the company undertook six research studies"*:
S. S. Vedula, L. Bero, R. W, Scherer, and K. Dickersin, Outcome reporting
in industry-sponsored trials of gabapentin for off-label use, *N Engl J Med*
361 (2009): 1963–1971 and supplementary appendix; S. S. Vedula, P. S.
Goldman, I. J. Rona, T. M. Greene, and K. Dickersin, Implementation of a
publication strategy in the context of reporting biases: A case study based on
new documents from Neurontin litigation, *Trials* 13 (2012): 136.

63 *"In the end, the company—now owned by Pfizer—agreed"*: G. Harris, Pfizer
to pay $430 million over promoting drug to doctors, *New York Times*, May
14, 2004, p. C1.

63 *"An extensive review turned up very few studies"*: R. Chou, Pharmacological
management of low back pain, *Drugs* 70 (2010): 387–402.

65 *"We have details of company decisions from employee interviews"*: M. Kimes, Bad
to the bone: A medical horror story, *Fortune*, October 8, 2012, http://features.
blogs.fortune.cnn.com/2012/09/18/synthes-norian-criminal/.

67 *"Digging a little deeper, newer research has challenged the value of vertebroplasty"*: D. F. Kallmes, B. A. Comstock, and P. J. Heagerty, et al., A randomized trial of vertebroplasty for osteoporotic spinal fractures, *N Engl J
Med* 361 (2009): 569–579; R. Buchbinder, R. H. Osborne, and P. R. Ebe-
ling, et al., A randomized trial of vertebroplasty for painful osteoporotic
vertebral fractures, *N Engl J Med* 361 (2009): 557–568.

7. Stabbed in the Back

69 *"After a nagging pain began in his right hip"*: The description of Groopman's
back problems was compiled from the following: J. Groopman, Prologue, in
Second Opinions (New York: Viking Penguin, 2000); J. Groopman, Exiting
a labyrinth of pain, chapter 6 in *The Anatomy of Hope* (New York: Random
House, 2004); J. Groopman, Surgery and satisfaction, chapter 7 in *How
Doctors Think* (Boston: Houghton Mifflin, 2007); J. Groopman, A knife in
the back, *New Yorker*, April 8, 2002; personal interview, May 10, 2013.

71 *"Surgery gives faster relief, but after a year or two"*: W. C. Peul, H. C. van
Houwelingen, and W. B. van den Hout, Surgery versus prolonged conser-
vative treatment for sciatica, *N Engl J Med* 356 (2007): 2245–2256; J. N.
A. Gibson and G. Waddell, Surgical interventions for lumbar disc prolapse,
Cochrane Database of Systematic Reviews, issue 2 (2007), art. no. CD001350,
doi:10.1002/14651858.CD001350.pub4; W. C. Jacobs, M. van Tulder, and
M. Arts, et al., Surgery versus conservative management of sciatica due to a
lumbar herniated disc: A systematic review, *Eur Spine J* 20 (2011): 513–522.

72 *"Consider the experience of another doctor, Sam Ho"*: R. Abelson and M. Petersen, An operation to ease back pain bolsters the bottom line, too, *New
York Times*, December 31, 2003.

73 *"Compared with removing part of a disc"*: R. A. Deyo, A. Nachemson, and S. K. Mirza, Spinal-fusion surgery—the case for restraint, *N Engl J Med* 350 (2004): 722–726.

74 *"Spine surgery shows some of the greatest variation among regions"*: R. A. Deyo and S. K. Mirza, Trends and variations in the use of spine surgery, *Clin Orthop Relat Res* 443 (2006): 139–146; Inpatient back surgery per 1,000 Medicare enrollees, by gender, *The Dartmouth Atlas of Health Care*, http://www.dartmouthatlas.org/data/table.aspx?ind=73&pf=1.

74 *"There were considerable differences of opinion among the surgeons"*: Z. N. Irwin, A. Hilibrand, M. Gustavel, R. McLain, W. Shaffer, M. Myers, J. Glaser, and R. A. Hart, Variation in surgical decision making for degenerative spinal disorders, Part I: Lumbar spine, *Spine* 30 (2005): 2208–2213.

74 *"He found that a decision to perform a fusion related more to surgeon preference"*: J. N. Katz, S. J. Lipson, R. A. Lew, L. J. Grobler, J. N. Weinstein, G. W. Brick, A. H. Fossel, and M. H. Liang, Lumbar laminectomy alone or with instrumented or noninstrumented arthrodesis in degenerative lumbar spinal stenosis: Patient selection, costs, and surgical outcomes, *Spine* 22 (1997): 1123–1131.

75 *"More recently, a neurosurgeon reported"*: N. E. Epstein, Are recommended spine operations either unnecessary or too complex? Evidence from second opinions, *Surgical Neurology International* 4 (2013): S353–S358.

75 *"The chair of orthopedic surgery"*: J. Yoo, Q & A response in *OHSU Health*, Spring 2013, p. 5.

77 *"Spinal instability is routinely given as a diagnosis"*: Groopman, Knife in the back.

77 *"One study directly compared fusion surgery with rehabilitation"*: J. I. Brox, O. Reikerås, Ø. Nygaard, et al., Lumbar instrumented fusion compared with cognitive intervention and exercises in patients with chronic back pain after previous surgery for disc herniation: A prospective randomized controlled study, *Pain* 122 (2006): 145–155.

78 *"Even so, by these criteria, the success rate of fusion surgery"*: S. Blumenthal, P. C. McAfee, and R. D. Guyer, et al., A prospective, randomized, multicenter Food and Drug Administration investigational device exemptions study of lumbar total disc replacement with the CHARITE artificial disc versus lumbar fusion, Part I: Evaluation of clinical outcomes, *Spine* 30 (2005): 1565–1575.

78 *"In another study, which examined a different fusion technique"*: J. Zigler, R. Delamarter, and J. M. Spivak, et al., Results of the prospective, randomized, multicenter Food and Drug Administration investigational device exemption study of the ProDisc-L total disc replacement versus circumferential fusion for the treatment of 1-level degenerative disc disease, *Spine* 32 (2007): 1155–1162.

78 *"In these studies, far fewer than half the patients return to work"*: T. H. Nguyen, D. C. Randolph, J. Talmage, P. Succop, and R. Travis, Long-term outcomes of lumbar fusion among workers' compensation subjects: A historical cohort study, *Spine* 36 (2011): 320–331; S. Maghout-Juratli, G. M. Franklin, S. K. Mirza, T. M. Wickizer, and D. Fulton-Kehoe, Lumbar fusion outcomes in Washington State workers' compensation, *Spine* 31 (2006): 2715–2723.

78 *"Consumer Reports surveyed almost one thousand readers"*: ConsumerReports. org, Relief for your aching back: What worked for our readers, March 2013, http://www.consumerreports.org/cro/2013/01/relief-for-your-aching-back/index.htm.

79 *"In large populations, this figure is almost one out of ten within two years"*: B. I. Martin, S. K. Mirza, B. A. Comstock, D. T. Gray, W. Kreuter, and R. A. Deyo, Reoperation rates following lumbar spine surgery and the influence of spinal fusion procedures, *Spine* 32 (2007): 382–387.

79 *"Over a seventeen-year time span, the number of fusion operations"*: HCUPnet, Agency for Healthcare Research and Quality, http://hcupnet. ahrq.gov/HCUPnet.jsp.

8. Surgical Gadgets and the Explosion of Fusion Surgery

81 *"In 2008, Arkansas neurosurgeon Patrick Chan pleaded guilty to taking kick-backs"*: The story of Dr. Chan was compiled from A. Dembner, Plea bolsters kickback case against Mass. medical firm, *Boston Globe,* January 4, 2008; L. Satter, Doctor pleads guilty to taking kickback; He also is to pay $1.5 million in civil suit, *ArkansasOnline,* January 4, 2008; news release, U.S. Attorney's Office, Eastern District of Arkansas, April 3, 2008.

82 *"Sure enough, in 2012, Orthofix International agreed to a $32 million settlement"*: D. Jeffrey, J. Feeley, and M. C. Fisk, Orthofix will pay U.S. $30 million to settle kickbacks, *Bloomberg News,* November 2, 2012; K. Ritter, Orthofix paying $30M to settle kickbacks case, *Businessweek,* November 2, 2012.

83 *"Also in 2012, Orthofix agreed to pay $5 million to settle charges"*: Press release, U.S. Securities and Exchange Commission, SEC charges Orthofix International with FCPA violations, July 10, 2012, http://www.sec.gov/news/press/2012/2012-133.htm.

83 *"Recall that in 2006 Medtronic agreed to pay the federal government"*: R. Abelson, Medtronic will settle accusations on kickbacks, *New York Times,* July 19, 2006.

84 *"Then, in 2007, four other device manufacturers agreed to a $310 million settlement"*: B. J. Feder, Artificial-joint makers settle kickback case, *New York Times,* September 28, 2007.

84   *"But in 2009, Medtronic had about $3.5 billion in sales"*: J. Carreyrou and
     T. McGinty, Top spine surgeons reap royalties, Medicare bounty, *Wall Street
     Journal*, December 20, 2010.

84   *"The publisher of an orthopedic newsletter said of the $310 million"*:
     Feder, Artificial-joint makers settle kickback case.

84   *"Consistent with the kickback lawsuits, Rosen told a Senate committee"*: A.
     Weintraub, The doctor vs. device makers, *Bloomberg Businessweek Magazine*,
     May 7, 2008.

85   *"Spinal fusion surgery has soared in this country over the last two decades"*:
     HCUPnet, Agency for Healthcare Research and Quality, http://hcupnet.
     ahrq.gov/HCUPnet.jsp.

85   *"Instead, the most common reason for spinal fusions may also be the most contro-
     versial"*: S. S. Rajaee, H. W. Bae, L. E. Kanim, and R. B. Delamarter, Spinal
     fusion in the United States: Analysis of trends from 1998 to 2008, *Spine* 37
     (2012): 67–76.

85   *"Surgery for worn-out discs is controversial"*: S. K. Mirza and R. A. Deyo, Sys-
     tematic review of randomized trials comparing lumbar fusion surgery to non-
     operative care for treatment of chronic back pain, *Spine* 32 (2007): 816–823.

86   *"In the Medicare population, a surgeon might be paid $600"*: E. J. Carragee,
     The increasing morbidity of elective spinal stenosis surgery: Is it necessary?
     JAMA 303 (2010): 1309–1310.

86   *"The Wall Street Journal reported that pedicle screws cost less than $100"*:
     Carreyrou and McGinty, Top spine surgeons reap royalties.

86   *"Remember that neurosurgeon Edward Benzel thought"*: R. Abelson and M.
     Petersen, An operation to ease back pain bolsters the bottom line, too, *New
     York Times*, December 31, 2003.

86   *"In comparing the United States with other developed countries"*: D. C. Cher-
     kin, R. A. Deyo, J. D. Loeser, T. Bush, and G. Waddell, An international
     comparison of back surgery rates, *Spine* 19 (1994): 1201–1206.

86   *"Our research shows not only that fusion operations"*: R. A. Deyo, S. K. Mirza,
     and B. I. Martin, et al., Trends, major medical complications, and charges
     associated with surgery for lumbar spinal stenosis in older adults, *JAMA* 303
     (2010): 1259–1265.

86   *"It appears to increase the need for repeat surgery as well"*: R. A. Deyo, B.
     I. Martin, W. Kreuter, J. G. Jarvik, H. Angier, and S. K. Mirza, Revision
     surgery following operations for lumbar stenosis, *J Bone Joint Surg Am* 93
     (2011): 1979–1986.

86   *"A randomized trial comparing three types of fusion operations"*: P. Fritzell, O.
     Hägg, P. Wessberg, and A. Nordwall, Swedish Lumbar Spine Study Group,
     Chronic low back pain and fusion: A comparison of three surgical tech-
     niques; A prospective multicenter randomized study from the Swedish Lum-
     bar Spine Study Group, *Spine* 27 (2002): 1131–1141.

87   *"In fact, it's not clear whether artificial discs offer any advantage"*: S. Blumen-thal, P. C. McAfee, and R. D. Guyer, et al., A prospective, randomized, multicenter Food and Drug Administration investigational device exemptions study of lumbar total disc replacement with the CHARITE artificial disc versus lumbar fusion, Part I: Evaluation of clinical outcomes, *Spine* 30 (2005): 1565–1575; J. Zigler, R. Delamarter, and J. M. Spivak, et al., Results of the prospective, randomized, multicenter Food and Drug Administration investigational device exemption study of the ProDisc-L total disc replacement versus circumferential fusion for the treatment of 1-level degenerative disc disease, *Spine* 32 (2007): 1155–1162.

88   *"It soon achieved almost $1 billion per year in sales"*: H. M. Krumholz, E. J. Emanuel, B. Hodshon, and R. Lehman, A historic moment for open science: The Yale University Open Data access project and Medtronic, *Ann Intern Med* 158 (2013): 910–912.

88   *"Some studies suggested that men receiving InFuse"*: E. J. Carragee, E. L. Hur-witz, and B. K. Weiner, A critical review of rhBMP-2 trials in spinal surgery: Emerging safety concerns and lessons learned, *Spine J* 11 (2011): 471–491.

88   *"A review of FDA reports"*: Carragee, A critical review of rhBMP trials in spinal surgery.

88   *"To make a long story short, here are some of the committee's findings"*: Staff of the Committee on Finance, U.S. Senate, *Staff Report on Medtronic's Influence on InFuse Clinical Studies* (Washington, D.C.: U.S. Government Printing Office, 2012).

89   *"Both teams concluded that there was no clinical advantage"*: M. C. Sim-monds, J. V. Brown, M. K. Heirs, J. P. Higgins, R. J. Mannion, and M. A. Rodgers, et al., Safety and effectiveness of recombinant human bone morphogenetic protein-2 for spinal fusion: A meta-analysis of individual-participant data, *Ann Intern Med* 158 (2013): 877–889; R. Fu, S. Selph, M. McDonagh, K. Peterson, A. Tiwari, and R. Chou, et al., Effectiveness and harms of recombinant human bone morphogenetic protein-2 in spine fu-sion: A systematic review and meta-analysis, *Ann Intern Med* 158 (2013): 890–902.

89   *"Both teams concluded that earlier articles misrepresented"*: M. A. Rodgers, J. V. E. Brown, M. K. Heirs, et al., Reporting of industry funded study out-come data: Comparison of confidential and published data on the safety and effectiveness of rhBMP-2 for spinal fusion, *Br Med J* 346 (2013): f3981; also Fu et al., Effectiveness and harms of recombinant human bone morphoge-netic protein-2.

90   *"In an investigation of payments to surgeons"*: Carreyrou and McGinty, Top spine surgeons reap royalties.

91   *"A famous cancer surgeon once argued"*: B. H. Lerner, The annals of extreme surgery, *New York Times*, August 29, 2011.

91   *"As some colleagues argue"*: G. M. Anderson, D. Juurlink, and A. S. Detsky, Newly approved does not always mean new and improved, *JAMA* 299 (2008): 1598–1600.

9. The Pointed Search for Relief

93   *"Trigger point injections don't sound controversial"*: M. Osterweis, A. Kleinman, and D. Mechanic, eds., *Pain and Disability: Clinical, Behavioral, and Public Policy Perspectives*, Institute of Medicine Committee on Pain, Disability and Chronic Illness Behavior (Washington, D.C.: National Academy Press, 1987), pp. 198–199, 285–292.

94   *"In 2009, a British guideline panel completed a thorough review"*: P. Savigny, P. Watson, and M. Underwood, on behalf of the Guideline Development Group, Early management of persistent non-specific low back pain: Summary of NICE guidance, *Br Med J* 338 (2009): b1805.

94   *"When he failed to condemn the guidelines"*: Z. Kmietowicz, President of British Pain Society is forced from office over NICE guidance on low back pain, *Br Med J* 339 (2009): b3049.

95   *"Directors of the British National Institute for Health and Clinical Excellence"*: M. Rawlins and P. Littlejohns, NICE outraged by ousting of pain society president, *Br Med J* 339 (2009): b3028.

95   *"This panel's conclusion was the same as the British guideline panel's"*: R. Chou, S. J. Atlas, S. P. Stanos, and R. W. Rosenquist, Nonsurgical interventional therapies for low back pain: A review of the evidence for an American Pain Society clinical practice guideline, *Spine* 34 (2009): 1078–1093.

95   *"When the American Pain Society published its guideline, ASIPP responded"*: L. Manchikanti, S. Datta, and S. Gupta, et al., A critical review of the American Pain Society clinical practice guidelines for interventional techniques, Part 2: Therapeutic interventions, *Pain Physician* 13 (2010): E215–E264.

96   *"Yet even Dr. Manchikanti acknowledged"*: A. Pollack, Before a wave of meningitis, shots were tied to risks, *New York Times*, October 11, 2012.

96   *"As one example, our analysis of Medicare data"*: J. Friedly, L. Chan, and R. Deyo, Increases in lumbosacral injections in the Medicare population, 1994 to 2001, *Spine* 32 (2007): 1754–1760.

96   *"Then, from 2000 to 2011, there was another 168 percent increase"*: L. Manchikanti, F. J. E. Falco, and V. Singh, et al., Utilization of interventional techniques in managing chronic pain in the Medicare population: Analysis of growth patterns from 2000 to 2011, *Pain Physician* 15 (2012): E969–E982.

96   *"Dr. Seth Waldman, who performs spinal injections"*: J. Groopman, A knife in the back, *New Yorker*, April 8, 2002.

99 *"For trigger point injections, the panel concluded"*: R. Chou, J. D. Loeser, and D. K. Owens, et al., Interventional therapies, surgery, and interdisciplinary rehabilitation for low back pain: An evidence-based clinical practice guideline from the American Pain Society, *Spine* 34 (2009): 1066–1077.

100 *"Unfortunately, most of these studies failed to show a reduction in subsequent surgery"*: C. Armon, C. E. Argoff, J. Samuels, and M.-M. Backonja, Assessment: Use of epidural steroid injections to treat radicular lumbosacral pain; Report of the therapeutics and technology assessment subcommittee of the American Academy of Neurology, *Neurology* 68 (2007): 723–729.

100 *"When we examined these geographic variations"*: J. Friedly, L. Chan, and R. Deyo, Geographic variation in epidural steroid injection use in Medicare patients, *J Bone Joint Surg Am* 90 (2008): 1730–1737.

100 *"Like the American Pain Society, the American Academy of Neurology"*: Armon et al., Assessment: Use of epidural steroid injections.

100 *"Led by Dr. Manchikanti"*: Manchikanti et al., Critical review of the American Pain Society clinical practice guidelines.

100 *"Authors of the Pain Society guidelines subsequently pointed to erroneous statements"*: R. Chou, S. J. Atlas, J. D. Loeser, R. W. Rosenquist, and S. P. Stanos, Guideline warfare over interventional therapies for low back pain: Can we raise the level of discourse? *J Pain* 12 (2011): 833–839.

101 *"An independent review of ten international guidelines"*: S. Dagenais, A. C. Tricco, and S. Haldeman, Synthesis of recommendations for the assessment and management of low back pain from recent clinical practice guidelines, *Spine J* 10 (2010): 514–529.

101 *"Another review of the studies on injection"*: N. Henschke, T. Kuijpers, S. M. Rubinstein, et al. Injection therapy and denervation procedures for chronic low-back pain: a systematic review, *Eur Spine J* 19 (2010): 1425–1449.

101 *"A more recent commentary concluded"*: J. B. Staal, P. J. Nelemans, and R. A. de Bie, Spinal injection therapy for low back pain, *JAMA* 309 (2013): 2439–2440.

101 *"In September 2012, Tennessee public health officials reported"*: M. A. Kainer, D. R. Reagan, and D. B. Nguyen, et al., Fungal infections associated with contaminated methylprednisolone in Tennessee, *N Engl J Med* 367 (2012): 2194–2203.

101 *"By July 2013, the U.S. Centers for Disease Control reported"*: Centers for Disease Control and Prevention, Multistate meningitis outbreak—current case count, July 1, 2013, http://www.cdc.gov/hai/outbreaks/meningitis-map-large.html.

102 *"One of these side effects is osteoporosis"*: A. Al-Shoha, D. S. Rao, J. Schilling, E. Peterson, and S. Mandel, Effect of epidural steroid injection on bone mineral density and markers of bone turnover in postmenopausal women, *Spine* 37 (2012): E1567–E1571.

102 *"Along with this, there appeared to be an increased risk"*: S. Mandel, J. Schilling, E. Peterson, D. S. Rao, and W. Sanders, A retrospective analysis of vertebral body fractures following epidural steroid injections, *J Bone Joint Surg Am* 95 (2013): 961–964.

10. Why Would You Get Better after Useless Therapy?

105 *"It turns out that improvement after about a year"*: H. Vastamaki, J. Kettunen, and M. Vastamaki, The natural history of idiopathic frozen shoulder: a 2- to 27-year followup study, *Clin Orthop Relat Res* 470, no. 4 (2012): 1133–1143.

105 *"Years ago, NBA basketball star Isaiah Thomas injured his back"*: K. Richardson, Thomas gives Pistons an unexpected spark and the Lakers fizzle, *Seattle Post-Intelligencer*, June 15, 1988.

106 *"In a pair of studies almost ten years apart"*: J. Coste, G. Delecoeuillerie, and A. Cohen de Lara, et al., Clinical course and prognostic factors in acute low back pain: An inception cohort study in primary care practice, *Br Med J* 308 (1994): 577–580; J. Coste, G. Lefrancois, and F. Guillemin, et al., Prognosis and quality of life in patients with acute low back pain: Insights from a comprehensive inception cohort study, *Arthritis Rheum* 51 (2004): 168–176.

106 *"Even in studies that included people with a longer duration"*: L. H. M. Pengel, R. D. Herbert, C. G. Maher, and K. M. Refshauge, Acute low back pain: Systematic review of its prognosis, *Br Med J* 327 (2003): 323.

106 *"Consider these expert pronouncements"*: J. Zimmerman, *The Diagnosis and Misdiagnosis of Back Pain* (Brunswick, Maine: Biddle Publishing Co., 1991), pp. 8–9.

108 *"To simulate a minor surgical procedure"*: J. B. Moseley, K. O'Malley, N. J. Petersen, T. J. Menke, B. A. Brody, D. H. Kuykendall, J. C. Hollingsworth, C. M. Ashton, and N. P. Wray, A controlled trial of arthroscopic surgery for osteoarthritis of the knee, *N Engl J Med* 347 (2002): 81–88.

108 *"Placebos probably don't work to save lives"*: A. Hrobjartsson and P. C. Gotzsche, Is the placebo powerless? An analysis of clinical trials comparing placebo with no treatment, *N Engl J Med* 344 (2001): 1594–1602.

108 *"But in some studies, 85 percent of subjects"*: J. A. Turner, R. A. Deyo, J. D. Loeser, M. Von Korff, and W. E. Fordyce, The importance of placebo effects in pain treatment and research, *JAMA* 271 (1994): 1609–1614.

108 *"Despite being well educated, trained in medicine"*: B. Blackwell, S. S. Bloomfield, and C. R. Buncher, Demonstration to medical students of placebo responses and non-drug factors, *Lancet* 1 (1972): 1279–1282.

108 *"And placebos have some surprising properties"*: R. L. Waber, B. Shiv, Z. Carmon, and D. Ariely, Commercial features of placebo and therapeutic efficacy, *JAMA* 299 (2008): 1016–1017; Turner et al., Importance of placebo effects.

108 *"It may be that the placebo effects of physical treatments"*: T. J. Kaptchuk, W. B. Stason, and R. B. Davis, et al., Sham device v inert pill: Randomised controlled trial of two placebo treatments, *Br Med J* 332, no. 7538 (2006): 391–397; T. J. Kaptchuk, P. Goldman, D. A. Stone, and W. B. Stason, Do medical devices have enhanced placebo effects? *J Clin Epidemiol* 53 (2000): 786–792.

109 *"In the 1950s, a popular minor operation"*: L. A. Cobb, G. I. Thomas, D. H. Dillard, K. A. Merendino, and R. A. Bruce, An evaluation of internal-mammary-artery ligation by a double-blind technic, *N Engl J Med* 260 (1959): 1115–1118.

109 *"But back in the 1970s, before we had modern imaging"*: E. V. Spangfort, The lumbar disc herniation: A computer-aided analysis of 2504 operations, *Acta Orthop Scand* 142, Suppl (1972): 1–95.

109 *"Just as an aside, that 40 percent success rate"*: S. Blumenthal, P. C. McAfee, and R. D. Guyer, et al., A prospective, randomized, multicenter Food and Drug Administration investigational device exemptions study of lumbar total disc replacement with the CHARITE artificial disc versus lumbar fusion, Part I: Evaluation of clinical outcomes, *Spine* 30 (2005): 1565–1575; J. Zigler, R. Delamarter, and J. M. Spivak, et al., Results of the prospective, randomized, multicenter Food and Drug Administration investigational device exemption study of the ProDisc-L total disc replacement versus circumferential fusion for the treatment of 1-level degenerative disc disease, *Spine* 32 (2007): 1155–1162.

109 *"One factor seems to be the important effect of expectations"*: Turner et al., Importance of placebo effects.

110 *"For example, the benefits of greater attention"*: M. A. Posternak and M. Zimmerman, Therapeutic effect of follow-up assessments on antidepressant and placebo response rates in antidepressant efficacy trials, *Br J Psych* 190 (2007): 287–292.

110 *"In a study of acupuncture"*: T. J. Kaptchuk, J. M. Kelley, and L. A. Conboy, et al., Components of placebo effect: Randomised controlled trial in patients with irritable bowel syndrome, *Brit Med J* 336, no. 7651 (2008): 999–1003.

111 *"Research has now thoroughly discredited many formerly standard treatments"*: R. Chou and L. H. Huffman, Nonpharmacologic therapies for acute and chronic low back pain: A review of the evidence for an American Pain Society/American College of Physicians Clinical Practice Guideline, *Ann Intern Med* 147 (2007): 492–504.

111 *"Earlier I described our study of transcutaneous electrical nerve stimulation"*: R. A. Deyo, N. E. Walsh, and D. C. Martin, et al., A controlled trial of transcutaneous electrical nerve stimulation (TENS) and exercise for chronic low back pain, *N Engl J Med* 322 (1990): 1627–1634.

112 *"Another example came from our study of bed rest for back pain"*: R. A. Deyo, A. K. Diehl, and M. Rosenthal, How many days of bed rest for acute low back pain? A randomized clinical trial, *N Engl J Med* 315 (1986): 1064–1070.

11. Manipulating the Pain

113 *"Chiropractors called a medical editor"*: J. H. Donahue, Morris Fishbein, M.D.: The "medical Mussolini" and chiropractic, *Chiropr Hist* 16, no. 1 (1996): 39–49.

113 *"The founder, D. D. Palmer, was a magnetic healer"*: J. B. Campbell, J. W. Busse, and H. S. Injeyan, Chiropractors and vaccination: A historical perspective, *Pediatrics* 105 (2000): 43, doi:10.1542/peds.105.4.e43, http://pediatrics.aappublications.org/content/105/4/e43.full.

114 *"Various theories focus on the small facet joints"*: W. C. Meeker and S. Haldeman, Chiropractic: A profession at the crossroads of mainstream and alternative medicine, *Ann Intern Med* 136 (2002): 216–227.

114 *"As an aside, osteopathy also originated in the late 1800s"*: American Association of Colleges of Osteopathic Medicine, History of osteopathic medicine, http://www.aacom.org/about/osteomed/Pages/History.aspx.

115 *"The public speaks with its feet"*: ConsumerReports.org, Relief for your aching back: What worked for our readers, March 2013, http://www.consumerreports.org/cro/2013/01/relief-for-your-aching-back/index.htm.

116 *"Fifteen years ago, I worked with Dr. Cherkin"*: D. C. Cherkin, R. A. Deyo, M. Battie, J. Street, and W. Barlow, A comparison of physical therapy, chiropractic manipulation, and provision of an educational booklet for the treatment of patients with low back pain, *N Engl J Med* 339 (1998): 1021–1029.

117 *"Like chiropractic adjustment, osteopathic adjustment appears to offer modest benefits"*: G. B. J. Andersson, T. Lucente, A. M. Davis, R. E. Kappler, J. A. Lipton, and S. Leurgans, A comparison of osteopathic spinal manipulation with standard care for patients with low back pain, *N Engl J Med* 341 (1999): 1426–1431; J. C. Licciardone, D. E. Minotti, R. J. Gatchel, C. M. Kearns, and K. P. Singh, Osteopathic manual treatment and ultrasound therapy for chronic low back pain: A randomized controlled trial, *Ann Fam Med* 11 (2013): 122–129.

117 *"An advantage of spinal manipulation is relative safety"*: Meeker and Haldeman, Chiropractic.

118 *"For example, we've used toothpicks in some research projects"*: K. J. Sherman, C. J. Hogeboom, D. C. Cherkin, and R. A. Deyo, Description and validation of a noninvasive placebo acupuncture procedure, *J Altern Complement Med* 8 (2002): 11–19.

118 *"With Dan Cherkin and his colleague Karen Sherman"*: D. C. Cherkin, K. J. Sherman, and A. L. Avins, et al., A randomized trial comparing acupuncture, simulated acupuncture, and usual care for chronic low back pain, *Arch Intern Med* 169 (2009): 858–866.

118 *"Well-designed studies from Germany"*: M. Haake, H. H. Muller, and C. Schade-Brittinger, et al., German acupuncture trials (GERAC) for chronic low back pain: Randomized, multicenter, blinded, parallel-group trial with 3 groups, *Arch Intern Med* 167 (2007): 1892–1898; B. Brinkhaus, C. M. Witt, and S. Jena, et al., Acupuncture in patients with chronic low back pain: A randomized controlled trial, *Arch Intern Med* 166 (2006): 450–457.

119 *"Finally, a recent study combined data"*: A. J. Vickers A. M. Cronin, and A. C. Maschino, et al., Acupuncture for chronic pain: Individual patient data analysis, *Arch Intern Med* 172 (2012): 1444–1453.

119 *"Functional MRI studies and hormone measurements"*: H. MacPherson, G. Green, and A. Nevado, et al., Brain imaging of acupuncture: Comparing superficial with deep needling, *Neurosci Lett* 434 (2008): 144–149; I. Lund and T. Lundeberg, Are minimal, superficial or sham acupuncture procedures acceptable as inert placebo controls? *Acupunct Med* 24 (2006): 13–15.

119 *"Other brain imaging studies suggest that true acupuncture"*: B. M. Berman, H. M. Langevin, C. M. Witt, and R. Dubner, Acupuncture for chronic low back pain, *N Engl J Med* 363 (2010): 454–461.

119 *"Surveys suggest that serious complications occur"*: Berman et al., Acupuncture for chronic low back pain.

119 *"Once again, Drs. Cherkin, Sherman, colleagues"*: D. C. Cherkin, K. J. Sherman, J. Kahn, R. Wellman, A. J. Cook, E. Johnson, J. Erro, K. Delaney, and R. A. Deyo, A comparison of the effects of 2 types of massage and usual care on chronic low back pain: A randomized, controlled trial, *Ann Intern Med* 155 (2011): 1–9.

120 *"A small number of other randomized trials"*: A. D. Furlan, M. Imamura, T. Dryden, and E. Irvin, Massage for low-back pain, *Cochrane Database of Systematic Reviews*, issue 4 (2008), art. no. CD001929.

120 *"These guidelines judged spinal manipulation"*: R. Chou, A. Qaseem, V. Snow, D. Casey, J. T. Cross, P. Shekelle, and D. K. Owens for the Clinical Efficacy Assessment Subcommittee of the American College of Physicians and the American College of Physicians/American Pain Society Low Back Pain Guidelines Panel, Diagnosis and treatment of low back pain: A joint clinical practice guideline from the American College of Physicians and the American Pain Society, *Ann Intern Med* 147 (2007): 478–491.

120   *"Another systematic review"*: A. D. Furlan, F. Yazdi, and A. Tsertsvadze, et al., Complementary and alternative therapies for back pain II, *Evid Rep Technol Assess* (Full Rep) 194 (2010): 1–764.

12. Nobody Takes It Seriously!

123   *"Pain evolved as a warning system, to alert us to the risk of tissue damage"*: Much of this discussion is compiled from Institute of Medicine, Introduction to *Relieving Pain in America: A Blueprint for Transforming Prevention, Care, Education, and Research* (Washington, D.C.: National Academies Press, 2011); A. Louw, I. Diener, D. S. Butler, and E. J. Puentedura, The effect of neuroscience education on pain, disability, anxiety, and stress in chronic musculoskeletal pain, *Arch Phys Med Rehabil* 92 (2011): 2041–2056.

123   *"Even a recent study reflected this problem"*: B. Darlow, A. Dowell, G. D. Baxter, F. Mathieson, M. Perry, and S. Dean, The enduring impact of what clinicians say to people with low back pain, *Ann Fam Med* 11 (2013): 527–534.

124   *"Furthermore, when nerve impulses arrive in the brain, they don't stimulate just one spot"*: A. Gawande, The pain perplex, *New Yorker*, September 21, 1998, pp. 86–94.

125   *"Very recent research, using highly specialized brain imaging"*: A. R. Mansour, M. N. Baliki, and L. Huang et al., Brain white matter structural properties predict transition to chronic pain, *Pain* 154 (2013): 2160–2168.

125   *"In fact, functional MRI is already revealing"*: C. Sprenger, F. Eippert, J. Finsterbusch, U. Bingel, M. Rose, and C. Büchel, Attention modulates spinal cord responses to pain, *Curr Biol* 22 (2012): 1019–1022; S. J. Bantick, R. G. Wise, and A. Ploghaus, et al., Imaging how attention modulates pain in humans using functional MRI, *Brain* 125 (2002): 310–319.

125   *"Recent studies, for example, suggest that persistent neck pain"*: A. V. Bortsov, J. E. Smith, and L. Diatchenko, et al., Polymorphisms in the glucocorticoid receptor co-chaperone FKBP5 predict persistent musculoskeletal pain after traumatic stress exposure, *Pain* 154 (2013): 1419–1426.

126   *"But in the long term, they may actually increase the problem of central sensitization"*: J. Mao, Opioid-induced abnormal pain sensitivity: Implications in clinical opioid therapy, *Pain* 100 (2002): 213–217; L. F. Chu, M. S. Angst, and D. Clark, Opioid-induced hyperalgesia in humans: Molecular mechanisms and clinical considerations, *Clin J Pain* 24 (2008): 479–495.

126   *"Here's a scenario that may be familiar to some people with persistent pain"*: A. J. Mariano, Patient chronic pain education: Taking self-management from the classroom to the clinic, VA Puget Sound Health Care System, Seattle,

http://www.hsrd.research.va.gov/for_researchers/cyber_seminars/archives/sopm-050112.pdf.

127 *"As a doctor-blogger writes"*: M. Kirsch, Accepting reasonable expectations is a gamechanger for patients, KevinMD.com, April 29, 2013, http://www.kevinmd.com/blog/2013/04/accepting-reasonable-expectations-gamechanger-patients.html.

129 *"Cognitive-behavioral therapy isn't traditional psychotherapy"*: R. J. Gatchel and K. H. Rollings, Evidence-informed management of chronic low back pain with cognitive behavioral therapy, *Spine J* 8 (2008): 40–44.

129 *"Some health care systems are experimenting with telephone versions"*: B. F. Dear, N. Titov, and K. N. Perry, et al., The Pain Course: A randomized controlled trial of a clinician-guided Internet-delivered cognitive behaviour therapy program for managing chronic pain and emotional well-being, *Pain* 154 (2013): 942–950; J. McBeth, G. Prescott, and G. Scotland, et al., Cognitive behavior therapy, exercise, or both for treating chronic widespread pain, *Arch Intern Med* 172 (2011): 48–57.

130 *"But see here: dozens of randomized trials have shown benefits"*: N. Henschke, R. W. J. G. Ostelo, and M. W. van Tulder, et al., Behavioural treatment for chronic low-back pain, *Cochrane Database of Systematic Reviews*, issue 7 (2010), art. no. CD002014.

130 *"In fact, it appears that this combination of cognitive-behavioral therapy and exercise"*: M. Monticone, S. Ferrante, B. Rocca, P. Baiardi, F. Dal Farra, and C. Foti, Effect of a long-lasting multidisciplinary program on disability and fear-avoidance behaviors in patients with chronic low back pain: Results of a randomized controlled trial, *Clin J Pain* 29 (2013): 929–938; M. K. Nicholas, A. Asghari, and F. M. Blyth, et al., Self-management intervention for chronic pain in older adults: A randomised controlled trial, *Pain* 154 (2013): 824–835; S. K. Vong, G. L. Cheing, F. Chan, E. M. So, and C. C. Chan, Motivational enhancement therapy in addition to physical therapy improves motivational factors and treatment outcomes in people with low back pain: A randomized controlled trial, *Arch Phys Med Rehabil* 92 (2011): 176–183.

130 *"These are skills that are available to you after office hours"*: S. A. Berkowitz and M. H. Katz, Thinking our way to better treatments of chronic pain, *Arch Intern Med* 172 (2012): 10–11.

13. Boot Camp

131 *"Attorney Eric Stevens"*: J. N. Weinstein, A 45-year-old man with low back pain and a numb left foot, *JAMA* 280 (1998): 730–736.

132 *"In a follow-up article a year later"*: J. Daley and E. E. Hartman, A 45-year-old man with low back pain and a numb left foot, 1 year later, *JAMA* 281 (1999): 1540.

133 *"Like most patients who have undergone spinal fusions"*: J. Groopman, A knife in the back, *New Yorker*, April 8, 2002.

133 *"When my sons were in grade school"*: J. Groopman, Exiting a labyrinth of pain, chapter 6 in *The Anatomy of Hope* (New York: Random House, 2004).

133 *"After carefully reviewing Groopman's medical history"*: much of the history of Groopman's experience is compiled from Groopman, *Anatomy of Hope*.

137 *"For people with acute back pain"*: A. Malmivaara, U. Hakkinen, and T. Aro, et al., The treatment of acute low back pain—bed rest, exercises, or ordinary activity? *N Engl J Med* 332 (1995): 351–355; A. Faas, A. W. Chavannes, J. T. M. van Eijk, and J. W. Gubbels, A randomized, placebo-controlled trial of exercise therapy in patients with acute low back pain, *Spine* 18 (1993): 1388–1395.

137 *"For persistent back pain"*: M. van Middelkoop, S. M. Rubinstein, A. P. Verhagen, R. W. Ostelo, B. W. Koes, and M. W. van Tulder, Exercise therapy for chronic nonspecific low-back pain, *Best Pract Res Clin Rheumatol* 24 (2010): 193–204; C. Smith and K. Grimmer-Somers, The treatment effect of exercise programmes for chronic low back pain, *J Eval Clin Pract* 16 (2010): 484–491; P. Oesch, J. Kool, K. B. Hagen, and S. Bachmann, Effectiveness of exercise on work disability in patients with non-acute non-specific low back pain: Systematic review and meta-analysis of randomized controlled trials, *J Rehabil Med* 42 (2010): 193–205.

138 *"Research studies on stretching exercises"*: K. J. Sherman, D. C. Cherkin, R. D. Wellman, A. J. Cook, R. J. Hawkes, K. Delaney, and R. A. Deyo, A randomized trial comparing yoga, stretching, and a self-care book for chronic low back pain, *Arch Intern Med* 171 (2011): 2019–2026; A. M. Hall, C. Maher, P. Lam, M. Ferreira, and J. Latimer, Tai Chi exercise for treatment of pain and disability in people with persistent low back pain: A randomized controlled trial, *Arthritis Care & Res* 63 (2011): 1576–1583; H. Cramer, R. Lauche, H. Haller, and G. Dobos, A systematic review and meta-analysis of yoga for low back pain, *Clin J Pain* 29 (2013): 450–460; J. P. Woodman and N. R. Moore, Evidence for the effectiveness of Alexander Technique lessons in medical and health-related conditions: A systematic review, *Int J Clin Pract* 66 (2012): 98–112; P. W. M. Marshall, S. Kennedy, C. Brooks, and C. Lonsdale, Pilates exercise or stationary cycling for chronic nonspecific low back pain: Does it matter? A randomized controlled trial with 6-month follow-up, *Spine* 38 (2013): E952–E959.

138 *"Further, exercise seems to reduce the frequency of repeat back pain"*: B. K. L. Choi, J. H. Verbeek, W. W.-S. Tam, and J. Y. Jiang, Exercises for prevention of recurrences of low-back pain, *Cochrane Database of Systematic Reviews*, issue 1 (2010). art. no. CD006555.

138 *"Finally, studies show that cognitive-behavioral therapy plus exercise"*: M. Monticone, S. Ferrante, B. Rocca, P. Baiardi, F. Dal Farra, and C. Foti, Effect of a long-lasting multidisciplinary program on disability and fear-avoidance behaviors in patients with chronic low back pain: Results of a randomized controlled trial, *Clin J Pain* 29 (2013): 929–938; M. K. Nicholas, A. Asghari, and F. M. Blyth, et al., Self-management intervention for chronic pain in older adults: A randomised controlled trial, *Pain* 154 (2013): 824–835; S. K. Vong, G. L. Cheing, F. Chan, E. M. So, and C. C. Chan, Motivational enhancement therapy in addition to physical therapy improves motivational factors and treatment outcomes in people with low back pain: A randomized controlled trial, *Arch Phys Med Rehabil* 92 (2011): 176–183; J. McBeth, G. Prescott, and G. Scotland, et al., Cognitive behavior therapy, exercise, or both for treating chronic widespread pain, *Arch Intern Med* 172 (2012): 48–57.

139 *"In fact, several studies suggest that the benefits of exercise"*: A. F. Mannion, M. Muntener, S. Taimela, and J. Dvorak. 1999 Volvo Award Winner in Clinical Studies: A randomized clinical trial of three active therapies for chronic low back pain, *Spine* 24 (1999): 2435–2448; A. F. Mannion, F. Caporaso, N. Pulkovski, and H. Sprott, Spine stabilisation exercises in the treatment of chronic low back pain: A good clinical outcome is not associated with improved abdominal muscle function, *Eur Spine J* 21 (2012): 1301–1310.

140 *"My colleague Donald Patrick and I coined the term"*: R. A. Deyo and D. L. Patrick, *Hope or Hype: The obsession with Medical Advances and the High Cost of False Promises* (New York: AMACOM, 2005).

14. Amplifying Your Voice

145 *"Studies suggest that people who are most confident"*: K. R. Sepucha, A. Fagerlin, M. P. Couper, C. A. Levin, E. Singer, and B. J. Zikmund-Fisher, How does feeling informed relate to being informed? The DECISIONS survey, *Med Decis Making* 30, no. 5, Suppl (2010): 77S–84S.

145 *"Recent disclosures make it clear that the price may vary fourfold"*: J. Young and C. Kirkham, Hospital prices no longer secret as new data reveals bewildering system, staggering cost differences, *Huffington Post Business*, October 7, 2013, http://www.huffingtonpost.com/2013/05/08/hospital-prices-cost-differences_n_3232678.html?view=print&comm_ref=false; B. Meier, J. C. McGinty, and J. Creswell, Hospital billing varies wildly, government data shows, *New York Times,* May 8, 2013.

146 *"Some researchers have studied what happens in doctors' offices"*: C. H. Braddock, K. A. Edwards, N. M. Hasenberg, T. L. Laidley, and W. Levinson, Informed decision making in outpatient practice: Time to get back to basics, *JAMA* 282 (1999): 2313–2320.

147 *"What about information you find on the web"*: G. Eysenback, C. J. Powell, O. Kuss, and E. R. Sa, Empirical studies assessing the quality of health information for consumers on the World Wide Web: A systematic review, *JAMA* 287 (2002): 2691–2700; A. Risk and C. Petersen, Health information on the Internet: Quality issues and international initiatives, *JAMA* 287 (2002): 2713–2715.

147 *"How about the patient education brochures"*: A. Coulter, V. Entwistle, and D. Gilbert, Sharing decisions with patients: Is the information good enough? *Br Med J* 318 (1999): 318–322.

147 *"Journalists themselves acknowledge sometimes overstating"*: D. Shaw, Medical miracles or misguided media? *Los Angeles Times*, February 13, 2000, p. A1.

147 *"And medical researchers often abet this process"*: Shaw, Medical miracles or misguided media?

149 *"By 2012, there were some 115 randomized trials"*: D. Stacey, F. Legare, and N. F. Col, et al., Decision aids for people facing health treatment or screening decisions, *Cochrane Database of Systematic Reviews*, published online January 28, 2014, art. no. CD001431, doi:10.1002/14651858.CD001431.pub4.

150 *"Initial testing of the program"*: B. S. Spunt, R. A. Deyo, V. M. Taylor, K. M. Leek, H. I. Goldberg, and A. G. Mulley, An interactive videodisc program for low back pain patients, *Health Educ Res* 11 (1996): 535–541.

150 *"We then undertook a randomized trial"*: R. A. Deyo, D. C. Cherkin, J. Weinstein, J. Howe, M. Ciol, and A. G. Mulley, Involving patients in clinical decisions: Impact of an interactive video program on use of back surgery, *Med Care* 38 (2000): 959–969.

151 *"We found that patients had greater knowledge gains"*: E. A. Phelan, R. A. Deyo, D. C. Cherkin, J. N. Weinstein, M. A. Ciol, W. Kreuter, and J. F. Howe, Helping patients decide about back surgery: A randomized trial of an interactive video program, *Spine* 26 (2001): 206–211.

152 *"Perhaps someday we can move away from the passive concept"*: B. Moulton, P. A. Collins, N. Burns-Cox, and A. Coulter, From informed consent to informed request: Do we need a new gold standard? *J R Soc Med* 106 (2013): 391–394.

15. Some Policy Implications

153 *"Current trends in the treatment of back pain"*: J. N. Mafi, E. P. McCarthy, R. B. Davis, and B. E. Landon, Worsening trends in the management and treatment of back pain, *JAMA Intern Med* 173 (2013): 1573–1581; J. I. Ivanova, H. G. Birnbaum, and M. Schiller, et al., Real-world practice patterns, health-care utilization, and costs in patients with low back pain: The long road to guideline-concordant care, *Spine J* 11 (2011): 622–632; T. S. Carey, J. K. Freburger, G. M. Holmes, L. Castel, J. Darter, and R. Agans, et al.,

A long way to go: Practice patterns and evidence in chronic low back pain care, *Spine* 34 (2009): 718–724; R. A. Deyo, S. K. Mirza, J. A. Turner, and B. I. Martin, Overtreating chronic back pain: Time to back off? *J Am Board Fam Med* 22 (2009): 62–68.

153 *"There are many reasons why"*: D. E. Casey, Why don't physicians (and patients) consistently follow clinical practice guidelines? *JAMA Intern Med* 173 (2013): 1581–1583.

154 *"That is, many guidelines are written by specialists"*: S. L. Norris, B. U. Burda, H. K. Holmer, L. A. Ogden, R. Fu, L. Bero, H. Schünemann, R. Deyo, Author's specialty and conflicts of interest contribute to conflicting guidelines for screening mammography, *J Clin Epidemiol* 65 (2012): 725–733.

154 *"The Institute of Medicine has established new standards"*: R. Graham, M. Mancher, and D. M. Wolman, et al., eds., Committee on Standards for Developing Trustworthy Clinical Practice Guidelines, Board on Health Care Services, *Clinical Practice Guidelines We Can Trust* (Washington, D.C.: National Academies Press, 2011).

154 *"We saw that patients who got a spinal imaging test"*: D. Kendrick, K. Fielding, and E. Bentley, et al., Radiography of the lumbar spine in primary care patients with low back pain: Randomized controlled trial, *Br Med J* 322, no. 7283 (2001): 400–405.

155 *"Similarly, patients who are convinced they need opioids"*: A. Lembke, Why doctors prescribe opioids to known opioid abusers, *N Engl J Med* 367 (2012): 1580–1581.

155 *"New data systems that track prescriptions"*: R. A. Deyo, J. M. Irvine, L. M. Millet, T. Beran, N. O'Kane, D. A. Wright, D. McCarty, Measures such as interstate cooperation would improve the efficacy of programs to track controlled drug prescriptions, *Health Aff (Millwood)* 32 (2013): 603–613.

157 *"Similarly, insurance coverage for physical therapy and for talk"*: Institute of Medicine, *Relieving Pain in America: A Blueprint for Transforming Prevention, Care, Education, and Research* (Washington, D.C.: National Academies Press, 2011).

157 *"North Carolina Blue Cross recently imposed such limits"*: BlueCross BlueShield of North Carolina, Corporate medical policy: Lumbar spine fusion surgery, September 2010, https://www.bcbsnc.com/assets/services/public/pdfs/medicalpolicy/lumbar_spine_fusion_surgery.pdf.

158 *"We were able to compare surgery for workers' compensation patients"*: B. I. Martin, G. M. Franklin, R. A. Deyo, T. Wickizer, J. D. Lurie, and S. K. Mirza, How do coverage policies influence practice patterns, safety, and cost of initial lumbar fusion surgery? A population-based comparison of workers' compensation systems, *Spine J*, November 7, 2013, doi:10.1016/j.spinee.2013.08.018, epub ahead of print.

158 *"At a needle-exchange program"*: K. M. Peavy, C. J. Banta-Green, and S. Kingston, et al., "Hooked on" prescription-type opiates prior to using heroin: Results from a survey of syringe exchange clients, *J Psychoactive Drugs* 44 (2012): 259–265.

158 *"The National Survey on Drug Use and Health"*: B. M. Kuehn, SAMHSA: Pain medication abuse a common path to heroin; Experts say this pattern likely driving heroin resurgence, *JAMA* 310 (2013): 1433–1434.

160 *"With Brook Martin again leading the charge"*: B. I. Martin, M. M. Gerkovich, R. A. Deyo, K. J. Sherman, D. C. Cherkin, B. K. Lind, C. M. Goertz, and W. E. Lafferty, The association of complementary and alternative medicine use and health care expenditures for back and neck problems, *Med Care* 50 (2012): 1029–1036.

160 *"The FDA is the key federal agency that regulates drugs and medical devices"*: R. A. Deyo, Gaps, tensions, and conflicts in the FDA approval process: Implications for clinical practice, *J Am Board Fam Pract* 17 (2004): 142–149.

161 *"A former director of the entire FDA remarked"*: D. W. Feigal, S. N. Gardner, and M. McClellan, Ensuring safe and effective medical devices, *N Engl J Med* 348 (2003): 191–192.

162 *"As one example, the painkiller Darvon"*: D. Wilson, Darvon pulled from market by F.D.A, *New York Times*, November 19, 2010; R. L. Barkin, S. J. Barkin, and D. S. Barkin, Propoxyphene (dextropropoxyphene): A critical review of a weak opioid analgesic that should remain in antiquity, *Am J Ther* 13 (2006): 534–542; Miller RR. Propoxyphene: a review. *Am J Hosp Pharm* 34 (1977): 413–423; R. A. Moore, S. L. Collins, J. Edwards, S. Derry, and H. J. McQuay, Single dose oral dextropropoxyphene, alone and with paracetamol (acetaminophen), for postoperative pain, *Cochrane Database of Systematic Reviews* issue 1 (1999), art. no. CD001440. doi:10.1002/14651858. CD001.

163 *"But it's one that the courts have recently begun to weaken"*: M. M. Boumil, Off-label marketing and the first amendment, *N Engl J Med* 362 (2013): 103–105.

164 *"These agencies were eliminated"*: S. Perry, The brief life of the National Center for Health Care Technology, *N Engl J Med* 307 (1982): 1095–1100; B. Bimber and D. H. Guston, Introduction: The end of OTA and the future of technology assessment, *Technological Forecasting and Social Change* 54 (1997): 125–130.

165 *"Dr. Jack Wennberg, a prominent doctor and policy researcher"*: J. E. Wennberg, The more things change . . . : The federal government's role in the evaluative sciences, *Health Affairs*, June 25, 2003, W3-308–W3-310, doi:10.1377/hlthaff.w3.308.

166 *"Indeed, a prominent health journalist"*: G. Schwitzer, 7 words (and more) you shouldn't use in medical news, http://www.healthnewsreview.org/

toolkit/tips-for-understanding-studies/7-words-and-more-you-shouldnt-use-in-medical-news/.

166   *"A government-sponsored public service campaign"*: R. Buchbinder, Self-management education en masse: Effectiveness of the Back Pain: Don't Take It Lying Down mass media campaign, *Med J Aust* 189, no. 10, Suppl (2008): S29–S32.

168   *"In 2007, Washington State passed legislation"*: B. M. Kuehn, States explore shared decision-making, *JAMA* 301 (2009): 2539–2541.

168   *"One of the early demonstrations, at the Group Health Cooperative"*: D. Arterburn, R. Wellman, E. Westbrook, C. Rutter, T. Ross, D. McCulloch, M. Handley, C. Jung, Introducing decision aids at Group Health was linked to sharply lower hip and knee surgery rates and costs, *Health Aff (Millwood)* 3 (2012): 2094–2104.

170   *"This strategy was used by Medicare"*: A. Fishman, F. Marinez, K. Naunheim, et al., National Emphysema Treatment Trial Research Group, A randomized trial comparing lung-volume-reduction surgery with medical therapy for severe emphysema, *N Engl J Med* 348 (2003): 2059–2073.

170   *"Recall too that Medicare recently decided on a CED approach"*: Department of Health and Human Services, Centers for Medicare and Medicaid Services, Transcutaneous electrical nerve stimulation (TENS) for chronic low back pain (CLBP), *MLN Matters,* no. MM7836, December 4, 2012, http://www.cms.gov/Outreach-and-Education/Medicare-Learning-Network-MLN/MLNMattersArticles/downloads/MM7836.pdf.

INDEX